HYPNO

SLIM

i

Published by
Sunday Books
London
in association with
Peter Grose Ltd
Monmouth

Printed and bound in Great Britain for Sunday Books and Peter Grose Ltd by Cox & Wyman Ltd, Reading, Berks.

Cover design: Mark Lomas

British Library C.I.P.
A catalogue record for this book is
available from the British Library

ISBN 1-898-88501-X

HYPNO
SLIM

Paul McKenna
and Heather Kirby

Published by
Sunday Books
London

in association with
Peter Grose Ltd
Monmouth

How We Proved Hypno Slim Works

We wanted to test Hypno Slim on an ordinary group of overweight people. So Paul McKenna, the TV hypnotist, and Heather Kirby, *Sunday* Magazine's health editor, went to a small, picturesque village in the heart of England.

There they invited anyone worried about their weight to become the first people in the world to try this extraordinary experiment.

The place chosen was Broadbottom, where they are used to having their legs pulled about being fat.

Twelve volunteers accepted the challenge. They all sat in the front room of one of the villagers' houses while Paul put them into a trance. He carefully explained what he was about to do. Some were apprehensive, but he made them feel relaxed. They waited. It felt like five minutes. In fact, to their surprise, they were "under" for nearly half an hour. While they were hypnotised, Paul began the process of re-programming their unconscious minds so they would never need to over eat again.

Ten of the twelve subjects were impressed. Two resisted—and, significantly, they were the only ones who stopped the healthy eating programme almost immediately. All the others stuck with it and managed to lose weight.

But what is even better, they felt they had been introduced to a completely new way of life. Their eating—and drinking— habits were changed forever. They felt better, fitter, younger, more enthusiastic about life. They can now cope with stressful situations more successfuly than before.

Unbelievable? Impossible? They proved it works. And this book and tape package is your chance to let it work for you.

Paul gave each volunteer a Hypno Slim tape with instructions to listen to it every day. Heather Kirby gave them a diet plan to follow, lots of healthy new recipes to try and nutritional advice to transform their bad eating habits into good ones.

For five months, Heather Kirby went every week to the Broadbottom community centre to weigh each of the men and women involved in our Hypno Slim experiment, and monitor their progress. She constantly adjusted their diets to make up for nutritional deficiencies, or their different likes and dislikes as they followed the programme.

This book and tape are your chance to do the same. Paul McKenna's tape will hypnotise you and reprogramme your unconscious mind, just as it did for our Broadbottom slimmers. Heather Kirby's nutrition guide, lifestyle advice and healthy recipes in the book can do for you what they did for the good people of Broadbottom.

There are eight different personal stories for you to follow. They are recorded in detail, including the times our Broadbottom friends fought back from their lapses.

Our volunteers are ordinary folk who had all tried—and failed—to lose weight. They succeeded with Hypno Slim. So can you.

About The Authors

Paul McKenna

Over 100 million people around the world have now seen Paul McKenna's remarkable television and stage hypnosis show. His sympathetic style and charismatic personality have turned him into the world's best known hypnotist.

He has used hypnosis to help thousands of people to improve their personal best—from Olympic athletes to business men and women.

With this book and tape he has created a new programme to tackle the deep, unconscious causes of excess weight. It will help those who want a healthier lifestyle to achieve their goals comfortably, and enduringly.

Heather Kirby

As health editor of *Sunday*, the colour magazine of *News Of The World,* Heather Kirby's advice is followed by the largest newspaper and magazine audience in Britain, *Sunday's* 12 million readers.

She has written on health subjects for a wide range of national newspapers and magazines, and is the author of two books on health and beauty.

She lives in central London with two teenage children, two dogs and a cat.

Also by Paul McKenna
The Hypnotic World of Paul McKenna

Also by Heather Kirby
A New You: Beauty Handbook
The Bastards (with Teresa Gorman MP)
The Menopause and HRT

Contents

HOW TO USE THE HYPNO SLIM PROGRAMME

Before you do anything else, read this page!

Safety first. DO NOT PLAY THE HYPNO SLIM TAPE WHILE DRIVING A CAR, OR WHILE OPERATING MACHINERY.

Before you start reading this book, find a quiet place and a quiet moment, and listen to the tape. You will need to set aside about 50 minutes, and you will need to give it your full attention.

Remember, the key to Hypno Slim is the reprogramming of your unconscious mind, and that will be achieved only by listening and re-listening to the tape every day.

When you have listened to both sides of the tape right through, you can start reading the rest of this book. The book is a supplement to the tape. It will show you, through the example of our Broadbottom slimmers, that Hypno Slim really works—and works for people just like you.

The book will also help you with some slimming menus and non-fattening recipes. Finally, we have included a few simple exercises.

You don't have to read the book all at once. You can dip into it for ideas whenever you like. And you don't have to follow slavishly the eating programme of any of our Broadbottom slimmers. What matters is that you use the tape every day to re-programme your unconscious mind. After that, slimming will seem the most natural thing in the world.

Hypno Slim is NOT a substitute for medical or psychiatric treatment. If you are in any doubt, consult your doctor before starting the programme.

Introduction

R esearch has shown that hypnosis is the most powerful way to bring about personal change. In this Hypno Slim programme we have brought together the latest techniques of hypnotic recording, a top nutritionist and a life-change strategy that has already helped thousands of people.

With Hypno Slim you lose weight, and you can stay slim permanently—but this isn't just a diet. Hypno Slim works because you don't just eat differently, you *think* differently. With Hypno Slim you are re-programming your unconscious mind and releasing energy into your life so your whole lifestyle, and the way you see yourself, will change.

The way you used to live could be described as a system for maintaining your unwanted weight. Your new lifestyle is a way of maintaining your desired weight—and enjoying it.

Living in a lighter, fitter body means feeling different—all day long.

Many people have the experience of losing weight by sheer will power and then putting it all back on again—because they have not made an inner psychological adjustment to living comfortably and enjoyably at their new weight.

The wonderful thing about this Hypno Slim programme is that it helps you to make that adjustment and integrate the results into your own life.

You don't have to cope all on your own. The work you do listening to the tape and going into trance is preparation for that change. You will prepare to enjoy and use the extra energy you have and make the most of your enhanced sensitivity.

Each of us has a unique personal possibility of happiness as we make the most of our life—and having your body fit and healthy helps bring that about.

So follow all the instructions on the tape and in this booklet and you will not only lose weight but you will experience a profound change in your relationship to the whole world. You will find that you can react quite differently to the things that used to lead to excessive eating—you handle stress better and you will find you enjoy a more active lifestyle.

Some of these changes will come as a surprise to you—but they will all arise from your own personal response to the exercises and hypnotic suggestions I give you.

The unconscious mind includes the wisdom of your body, which is coded in the genes of every single one of our cells. The body knows how to operate efficiently and healthily: that knowledge is literally built into it. You will find that day by day you are able to pay more and more attention to the cues and signals of the body which guide your eating, sleeping and activity. You will become free from addictive eating cycles and from eating for emotional reasons.

You will discover that in this course you are asked to increase the amount of exercise in your daily life. For some people that is an instant turn off. The great thing about using hypnosis is that as you start taking the exercise you will soon find that your body will begin to give you positive feedback! You will find yourself liking things that you thought you'd never be able to do—let alone enjoy!

Your body has the wisdom to guide you to a more balanced lifestyle and help you to integrate an appropriate level of physical exercise into your life: all you have to learn to do is work with it, not against it.

For many people this amount of change sounds a bit daunting. *DON'T WORRY*—it will all happen quite naturally and gradually, and it will be guided and assisted by using the Hypno Slim tape. You've got a wonderful transformation to look forward to!

What you need to bring to this programme is Positivity, Motivation and Determination. The hypnotic trances work like magnifiers so, as you read this introduction and think "Yes, I want to lose weight," you are sowing a seed in your mind. In trance that thought is integrated into the world view that you unconsciously use when you make decisions, and each time you go into trance its effect on your world view and your habits increases.

You can use the tape as often as you wish, but the minimum you should use it is as follows:

Use side one of the tape every day for a week, then use it at least once a week after that to refresh your memory and re-charge your motivation. Use the hypnotic tape, side two, every day.

It is very exhilarating when you first really feel you are lighter, and can fit into smaller clothes sizes. KEEP USING THE HYPNOTIC TAPE DURING THIS TIME—your unconscious mind is still adjusting to running a lighter body. Even when you reach your target weight, keep using the tape. To make sure you stay at the new weight you desire, very many small but important habits need to have changed and each one makes the slight change in your everyday unconscious sense of self.

Don't be too impatient or too quick to finish—stay with the programme.

When you have maintained your ideal weight for a month you can use the tape less often. Cut down to three times a week, then twice a week, then once a week and then once a month. But if ever you feel anxious, or feel worried about food, use the tape again to reinforce your new lifestyle.

Now, to kick start your positive frame of mind, write down a list of ten reasons why you want to lose weight and ten things you want to do when you are slimmer. Write them out right now on a piece of card so that you can carry it around with you and look at it whenever you want, to remind yourself of where you are heading.

Of course you don't have to stop at ten: you can add to it whenever you want.

And now that you know where you are going, read on to find out about our Broadbottom slimmers—the people who proved it really is possible.

Each of them has a satisfying, healthy diet and they've lost weight. Read on, and listen to the tapes to start that process of permanent, healthy weight loss and become the new, healthier, happier you!

Paul McKenna
April, 1994

Who Is That Fat Freak? IT'S ME!

Dieting is all in the mind. Every slimmer knows that perfectly well. The problem is getting the message from brain to mouth. It may appear to be a short journey. After all, they're only a few centimetres apart.

Yet for most people who want to lose weight the distance might just as well be 10,000 miles because the way to shed pounds appears to be long, arduous and perilous. The majority of dieters will tell you they'd as soon try to climb the north face of the Eiger. And they'd have just as much chance of success.

That's why hypnosis is the answer to a dieter's prayer. And we're not talking here about those clever clogs who decide they are overweight, cut down on all the wrong things and emerge six weeks later slim, trim and pleased as punch with themselves. With will power like theirs, who needs help?

We're talking about the average overweight Brit who didn't notice he or she was getting bigger...and bigger...and bigger. The kind of people who are too busy to bother, having too much fun eating and drinking whatever they like to care, or who just don't look at themselves critically in the mirror often enough.

Suddenly they wake up one day and there they are: FAT.

It's sometimes a holiday snap that brings it all home. When you notice the donkey's face looks particularly glum as it bears your colossal bum beachwards.

Or a wedding photo taken when you're wearing your Sunday best and you thought you looked like the bees knees. Only to discover when the prints are handed back to you at the chemist's, the elephant on the end isn't somebody else's tubby relative. The bloater with the bulges is YOU.

It's a depressing discovery and where do you turn to for comfort? The biscuit tin. The chocolate box. The wine bottle. It's a familiar cycle to any dieter and one that is notoriously difficult to break. But our group of ordinary folk proved it can be done.

We chose the village of Broadbottom, near Manchester, because it is such a matchlessly apt name. And the villagers are good sports.

They are used to having their legs pulled and can take a joke about big bums with the best of them. The trouble is, it stops being so funny when your vital statistics begin to tot up to a figure that is far from amusing. Being seriously overweight is dangerous, they know that.

We also wanted a friendly group of neighbours who could get on together and encourage each other when the going got tough. And that's just what our slimmers from Broadbottom did. They entered into the spirit of the thing from the word go. They were prepared to work hard to show the world that they may be Broadbottom by name—but not by nature!

It isn't easy. They'd be the last to claim all you need to do is lie down and listen to the hypnotic words while your fat drains away. But what they have proved is that with help from hypnosis, you can change your attitude to food.

Turn on the tape when you go to bed and listen to the messages which will seep into your subconscious. You may fall asleep as many of our group did before the tape ends. That doesn't matter. Another day you will listen to a different section. You can pick up where you left off the previous night. What matters is that you listen to the tape regularly because it is very, very easy to forget. Funnily enough, it is often just as you are eating the last mouthful of a piece of chocolate cake that you remember you are supposed to be trying to lose weight. Haven't you found that? Odd, isn't it? But that's the mind, a weird and wonderful place where strange things happen. And that is why you have to retrain your mind before you can start tackling your body.

What the slimmers in Broadbottom did not do is Go On A Diet. To eat nothing but pineapple for five days or stuff yourself full of beans until you explode is no long-term solution for a lifetime's bad eating habits.

Diets just replace bad eating habits with daft eating habits. But with the help of hypnosis and the examples of our Broadbottom dieters, you will learn that eating, so long as it is healthy eating, is what makes you slim. And starving makes you fat.

The overweight people in Broadbottom never thought they would succeed—most of them have tried other diets. But they were keen to try hypnosis. This was something new, something sensational and what's more, it sounded as if it didn't need any will power. Dream on. That easy it isn't.

What they had to embark on was a partnership between the tape, Heather Kirby's healthy eating advice and a programme of exercises.

Naturally everyone just wants to listen to a tape, that's nice and effortless. Lie back and dream of treacle puddings and all your troubles disappear. Unfortunately for them—and you—there is more to the Hypno Slim plan than that. There is a lot of hard work ahead if you want to lose weight. The advantage this slimming programme has over all the others is that it teaches you how to eat and drink sensibly.

Let hypnosis work on your subconscious and you will be amazed at what a wonderfully clever person, someone who is keenly interested in nutrition and in curing minor ailments through healthy eating, you become.

It isn't healthy or clever to abuse your body by over-eating. There are enough illnesses and diseases lurking about which we can't avoid without us piling on the agony via biscuits and buns. Silly, isn't it, to invite trouble? Yet that's what many of us do. Some of us carry around the equivalent of two toddlers, putting unnecessary strain on our heart, lungs, muscles and joints.

But if you are determined enough to change your shape, hypnosis, eating the right foods and doing energetic exercise will make it happen. With our Hypno Slim programme, you will be learning how to change the habits of a lifetime.

The last thing you should think or talk about is being on a diet. Instead, approach the next few months as if you were on a course, making notes, checking facts, swotting up about nutrients, re-educating yourself.

Read how Janis, June, Brenda, David, Pauline, Andrew, Anne and Carol did it. They all lead different lives, they all have individual likes and dislikes and some of them are bound to match your own. From them you will learn how difficult it was at times, how they fell by the wayside occasionally, how they ditched all their good resolutions when they were celebrating someone's anniversary, or were strict with themselves and still didn't lose weight but how they kept going nevertheless.

What they ate will probably surprise you because it is so normal. The adjustments they had to make to their meals were not monumental. But neither does eating the odd biscuit with a cup of coffee seem so sinful. It's just that those little things add up to a lot when they turn themselves into fat deposits.

What our friends in Broadbottom had to do, constantly, was ask themselves a lot more questions about everything they were eating. Am I getting enough vitamin B? Is there any magnesium in my diet? How many meals based on pulses do we eat in a week? Should I cook this spinach or have it raw in a salad? Should I buy smaller dinner plates? Will the children take to ratatouille? How can I make myself drink all that water?

Once you start thinking about why you are eating what you are eating— and the hypnosis tape will help you to do that—the examples of our Broadbottom dieters will inspire you. They lost weight slowly over a period of six months, not six weeks. They were not sold a smart-alec solution to a difficult and serious problem but were given very careful guidance about a new way of enjoying food. It is a message which needs reinforcing all the time. Which is why you have to keep listening to the tape and follow all the instructions that make the effect stronger and stronger.

HOW TO CHECK YOUR CORRECT
HEIGHT/WEIGHT RATIO

The so-called desirable weight/height charts issued by insurance companies are not always the best guide to illustrate how overweight you are. Muscle weighs more than fat, for instance, so someone who does a lot of exercise could be heavier but trimmer. People are also built differently. A tall person who is carrying excess weight can get away with what a small person cannot. A better guide is the Body Mass Index. To work out yours, divide your weight in kilogrammes by the square of your height in metres. It's not as complicated as it sounds, but a calculator may help.

If you score under 25 you are OK, between 25-30 you are moderately overweight. If you score between 30-40 you are beginning to be obese and if you score more than 40 you are in serious trouble. Your health is very definitely at risk and you should take steps to do something about it immediately.

Here's how to work out your body mass: say you are 5ft 2ins (1.58 metres) and weigh 9stone 10lbs (59.9kg). You multiply 1.58 by 1.58 which gives you 2.49 and divide 59.9 by 2.49 which gives 24.05—just within the OK band.

THE TEN COMMANDMENTS

Copy this page out and pin it up somewhere you will read it every day—no one has a worse memory than a dieter!

1. Drastically cut consumption of saturated fats.
2. Ban from your life refined sugar and anything containing it.
3. Bump up your intake of fresh vegetables and pulses.
4. Eat at least one apple, pear, or kiwifruit every day.
5. Drink two litres of still water every day.
6. Stop smoking.
7. Gradually cut down coffee and tea intake.
8. Work up to at least 15 minutes strenuous exercise each day.
9. Switch to wholemeal everything.
10. Keep a seven-day diet diary occasionally.

Teacher's Torture

CAROL HULMES

Age: 43
Height: 5' 4"
Weight: 10 stone 11 lbs
Target: 9 stone
Weight so far: 8 stone 12 lbs

C arol is a primary school teacher, married with two children, aged 14 and 10. After a tiring day's teaching, Carol used to sit down and relax with a glass of wine. Unfortunately it didn't just stop at one glass: she ended up drinking at least half a bottle—or more.

That was before she joined our Hypno Slim experiment. Now she is a changed woman. Not only is she two stones lighter, she has given up her habitual tipple. And she has acquired a sexy new shape.

"The trouble is, my husband is often busy with his work during the week and is chairman of a rugby club which keeps him occupied some evenings and quite a few weekends. So I often feel lonely and I started to drink for company," said Carol.

"It began with the odd glass, then I started to put the bottle by the side of my armchair to save me having to get up and go to the kitchen until, unconsciously, it became a habit."

Carol, whose weight had gradually crept on when she was at college worrying about her exams, admits, "I had just not realised I'd become complacent, I just wasn't bothered about the way I looked. I was not even aware of it most of the time.

"I always assumed I was naturally on the chubby side, a plump person with big bones. When my children were born they were quite large and I presumed that was natural, given my own size, but now I realise I was mistaken."

Like so many overweight people, Carol had come to see food—and wine—as a source of comfort, a way to beat loneliness and stress. She needed to re-programme her unconscious mind into a healthier approach to food. And, with Hypno Slim, she succeeded.

Here's how Carol gained top marks:

She may not have been interested in what was happening to her body before but Carol was to become one of our most conscientious dieters. She listened to her hypnosis tape every day at first and then two or three times a week. She did daily work outs with exercise videos and stuck rigidly to her diet. It paid off.

Her drinking habit had to go. And not just because alcohol puts weight on, it can cause a lot of other problems. But since recent research shows that alcohol can also help clear the arteries to the heart, there is a genuine excuse for not eliminating it entirely from your life.

In Carol's case we suggested almost total abstinence until she reached her target weight. The only exception was her reward, two glasses of wine, every week after she had been particularly successful. The last thing we believe is that diets should be like purgatory; every slimmer needs treats to help keep them going.

"The more you have to lose the more you have to listen to the tape," Carol found. "I have lost more than I planned but I'm very happy with my shape now and I am concentrating on toning and strengthening my muscles. But I still listen to the tape two or three times a week.

"I think I probably always will because, although eating healthily has become a way of life, I'd hate to start backsliding. Being part of a group has helped because you don't want to let other members of the team down.

"I've gone down from a size 14 to a size 10 and I don't even feel as if I have been on a diet.

"The messages on Paul's tape are obviously getting through. He's right about saying my body knows best what is good for it. I have felt my body responding in a positive way—at no time did I feel 'deprived'. Paul's tape makes you re-think the whole concept of food and what it is for.

"This experience has been a re-education for me. I was not aware how much fat I was eating or which foods have fibres. What I thought was healthy eating was totally different to what I am eating now. We never ate lentils before, for instance, now it is a regular item two or three times a week. And I don't suppose I drank more than the odd glass of water, now

11

I drink nothing else. My son drinks gallons too, and he has a lovely complexion.

"My daughter is 14, just the right age to impress healthy eating habits on. The children seem to have taken to the vegetables I am now cooking quite naturally. They love all the courgette, spinach and tomato dishes I am making.

"Although I still cook a proper Sunday lunch with beef and Yorkshire pudding, I don't eat the meat or Yorkshire. My taste buds have changed completely and I just don't want meat any more.

"At lunchtime I have a sandwich followed by yoghurt or fresh fruit.

"When we go out to eat my favourite is Italian seafood. When we entertain at home I never make puddings, I will make a fish starter followed by something simple like beef stroganoff and have cheese and biscuits.

"Even at Christmas we didn't have pudding. And we didn't have mince pies either! My husband loves puddings so I bought individual ones for him, but the children and I couldn't manage it, not after all the other trimmings."

Of course, being a teacher Carol is used to discipline and, boy, did she need it. Two days after she started our Hypno Slim programme she was teaching a gymnastic class, landed badly and pulled the ligaments in her ankle.

But that didn't stop her getting on with the exercises she was able to do. Although skipping, walking and even swimming were out, she did lots of upper body, leg and hip exercises at home. And, as soon as she could walk properly again, joined a weekly aerobics and aquarobics class.

The inches started dropping off almost immediately. Every week you could see a difference in Carol's shape. From a body verging on the matronly, an athletic, healthy—and younger looking—woman began to emerge. First to slim down were her hips: they went from 39-1/2" to 37". Then she lost two inches from her bust but at that time her waist was still 28". It started to disappear later.

At the beginning, for one day a week, Carol either fasted or nearly fasted, which means eating just raw vegetables and maybe an apple in the evening. Torture for most people, but terrific for getting rid of toxins from the body.

At Sunday pub lunches she quickly learned to manage without alcohol: "Instead, I drank soda with ice and lemon and it was lovely. I didn't notice there was no gin or vodka in it."

At the Parent Teachers' Association meeting she drank soda water and, when one of her husband's customers invited them to a Chinese banquet, she suggested they turn it down—at least until she had reached her target. "I know I would have felt guilty just sitting there picking so I thought I was more sensible to put it off until later."

Even watching the rest of her family tuck into chips didn't worry her. "The great thing about this diet is I'm not hungry. I'm eating regularly and it's not like being on a diet. Because you have done it slowly, it becomes part of your life.

"Because you have stressed the benefits of having a proper breakfast, sometimes I will cook a real meal. I've invented a no-fat omelet with tomato, mushrooms, garlic and green pepper. I whip up an egg, pour it over and stick it in the microwave for a few minutes. It tastes delicious."

The secret of really successful slimming is to eat—but eat the right things.

You feel hungry? Eat. Have a drink of water first, then tuck into a crispbread and yeast extract, a low-cal soup, a plate of raw carrots, cauliflower and yellow peppers. Carol has made up a whole series of quick, healthy dishes like courgettes, tomatoes and garlic fried in a tiny dot of margarine then baked in the oven with a sprinkling of parmesan cheese on top.

Filling that gap doesn't have to mean a biscuit.

Carol also gave up putting salt in her food (no one in the family noticed the difference) and cut down her caffeine intake. Now she drinks two or three cups of Earl Grey tea a day. She also managed to drink her allowance of two litres of water and when children wanted biscuits, she bought them individual ones rather than a packet so she wouldn't be tempted.

She was also strict with the children when it came to her time for working out. "I made it a rule that under no circumstances was I to be disturbed, this was my hour and I was going to finish my exercises. If they were desperate for a drink they had to help themselves or wait.

"The same applied to homework and everything else. I gave them plenty of warning and told them what we were going to do together afterwards so they had no excuse for interrupting me. It's no use starting an exercise video then having to stop every five minutes. You have to keep going otherwise it doesn't do you as much good."

One of the great satisfactions of losing weight is seeing your friends' jaws drop or getting unfamiliar compliments. Carol also encountered another bonus. "When I go to the gym to join the aerobics class I feel like one of the gang now. Before, I always felt self-conscious because I was larger than everyone else. Now, also, I miss it if I don't go, my body seems to need the extra exercise."

Carol began to notice the weight dropping off her shoulders, upper arms and bust from about the second week. The hip bones which had been buried for years emerged later. "For me, having a hip bone is a new experience," she said. When she bought her first size 12 in years she cheered. When she bought her first size 10 skirt—and it was roomy—she wanted to wear it with the label on the outside.

"It's nice to know you can wear what you like, tight jodhpurs if you want. I feel far more attractive now and am getting more comments from my colleagues at work. We often go out for a meal or a drink together and I can't remember anyone passing a comment before but they do now. Someone even whistled at me the other day when I was wearing my new outfit."

A wolf-whistle may be politically incorrect but to a born-again slimmer woman it is a wonderful sound!

TEACHER'S TORTURE

Carol described herself before our experiment began as "not a breakfast person". But I persuaded her that doing without anything in the morning is unhealthy so she changed from having just a cup of tea to something more substantial.

Choose one from each of the following sections:

Breakfasts
All Bran
1 Wheatabix
Tesco's luxury Muesli (it has no fattening nuts)
3 eggs a week, sometimes cooked with vegetables
Smoked haddock, 1 slice granary bread soaked with juice from fish
Prunes, Bran Flakes and plain yoghurt

Light meals
Sandwiches: two slices wholemeal bread with no butter or spread, a dot of low cal mayonnaise (sometimes) with lean corned beef and fresh beetroot, or
Tuna and cucumber, or

Cottage cheese and salad, or

Smoked salmon, cottage cheese and celery, or

Grilled lean bacon with grilled tomato

One slice toast, 2 grilled sardines, lemon juice and black pepper

Cooked spinach with cottage cheese, grilled

Wholemeal toast, Edam cheese, mustard, tomato, grilled

Small smoked mackerel, salad of lettuce, tomatoes and orange

Main Meals

Jacket potato with cottage cheese and pineapple or low-sugar baked beans

Lemon sole, sweet corn, broad beans

Steamed salmon with parsley sauce and mashed potato, peas and sweet corn

Steamed fish, summer cabbage, new potatoes, grilled tomatoes

Roast breast of chicken, jacket potato, cottage cheese, pineapple and fresh tomato

Macaroni, Edam cheese, American smoked ham, spring onions baked with tomatoes on top

Peppered mackerel, side salad, 1 slice wholemeal bread

Poached trout with broccoli

Chicken breast, marinated in plain yoghurt and tandoori powder, served with brown rice or wholemeal pasta

B-B-Q chicken, nan bread, salad

No-fat omelet

Spaghetti with mixed seafood in tomato and garlic sauce, ready cooked with squid, prawns, mussels and cockles

Snacks

Low calorie yoghurts

Fruit (Carol cut down drastically on bananas)

Drinks (one per meal)

Tomato or grapefruit juice

Earl Grey tea

Plus 2 litres water daily

Treats (one a week)

2 glasses wine

Indian takeaway

Farmer's Fare

JANIS PRYCE

Age: 43
Height: 5' 4"
Weight: 13 stone
Target: 10 stone
Weight so far: 10 stone 2lbs

J anis is a farmer's wife with three children: a daughter of 21 and sons aged 18 and 14. She is a wonderful cook who bakes delicious cakes for her relatives and friends in the village. If someone is getting married or has a special birthday or anniversary to celebrate, Janis makes the cake.

"And unfortunately I have a sweet tooth," she told us. "I could never go on a fast and would even find a diet difficult. What I want to do is eat the same as I eat now but less of it."

That, if what you eat is healthy to begin with, is the best "diet" of all. It means you don't have to go out and buy special foods. And you don't have to suffer in silence while your family eats the lovely meal you have prepared while you pick at rabbit fare.

Janis knows herself. "I'd just binge if I went on a diet," she admitted. "If I had to buy special slimming things I'd make myself miserable.

Janis's mother is overweight, so she takes after her, and her younger son has the same build. "But he is so active he isn't fat like me," she says.

Like the vast majority of us, Janis was brought up to finish everything on her plate. "That's something I'll never be able to get out of so the only answer is to put less on in the first place."

Like all dieters, Janis needed to adjust her unconscious mind's approach to eating. While food can and should always bring pleasure, she had allowed her unconscious mind to associate over-eating with good times.

She listened to the Hypno Slim tape and began the Hypno Slim programme.

Here's how she fared:

Janis has continued to eat with her family and although I suggested she use a smaller size plate—sometimes it is something as simple as that which can get you out of the habit of over-eating—she decided not to. "I didn't want to make me different from the rest of them, I didn't want to be conscious that I was on a diet. But I don't put as much food on my plate as I used to, only about half as much."

Now, instead of the usual generous portions of potential fatteners like homemade apple pie, Janis has retrained her stomach to be content with a finger-sized piece.

That, she is convinced, is thanks to the hypnosis. "Before, I was always shovelling large pieces of cake or pudding down me, now I am aware of what I am doing and stop."

Janis was intrigued by the hypnosis. "I was conscious all the time I was being hypnotised. I didn't feel as if I was under any sort of power but at the same time I couldn't move," she said.

"It's really interesting and must have helped because I have completely changed my eating habits and don't feel deprived or depressed about eating less. That isn't to say I haven't fallen by the wayside once or twice but nothing like I used to when I went on a diet—and I have tried several.

"I try to plan at least one meal ahead because I tend to pick when I'm hungry. But if I know what's coming next, I find it easier not to eat. I don't go in for cooking anything particularly slimming but I do attempt to cut down on fattening things where I can. For instance, I will make a pie with the crust only on top, not the bottom as well. Or substitute pastry for a crumble of wholemeal breadcrumbs mixed with herbs. And if I make a cheese and onion pie I will make it with low fat cheddar and serve it with a green salad."

Janis came to one of our weekly weigh-ins with guilt written all over her face. The tale of the liquorice humbugs is one, with slight variations, which will be familiar to everyone who has ever tried to lose weight. There is always some evil "friend" who says, "Oh, just have the one, it won't do you any harm. You're not fat, anyway." Don't you love them? Janis's friend had been on a visit to a factory where they make liquorice humbugs and, of course, generously presented Janis with a jumbo-size bag. "I could no more throw them away or ration myself to two a week than fly. I ate them and ate them until I was nearly sick," she admitted. "When they were gone I actually cheered!"

Before her hypnosis session and our healthy eating plan, Janis thought nothing of eating a packet of crisps while having a drink before going out for an evening meal. And, like most who took up our challenge, she hardly ever had any water to drink.

"I still have difficulty getting through two litres a day and can't drink it cold from the fridge," she says. "But I am trying. What I find frustrating about the diet is feeling guilty if we have an alcoholic drink. I wish I didn't have to worry about it."

She won't, of course, once her weight has dropped to ten stone and she has kept it there for a year. So long as the odd shared bottle of wine doesn't become a nightly habit, she will be able to drink and enjoy it without that guilty feeling.

One drinking habit Janis has acquired is for fruit teas. When her husband Charles makes his usual request to "Put the kettle on" in the past that automatically meant a cup of tea. "Now I choose from a selection of blackcurrant, raspberry, apple or orange teas and I have cut out having a biscuit altogether because that is one of the things I was eating but not needing. The teas are much more refreshing than I thought they'd be, much more thirst quenching."

Another switch Janis has made is to a low-cal chocolate drink at bedtime. "Now I have a drink with only 40 calories in it and, although it says on the tin two heaped teaspoons, I find that one is more than enough." That, as anyone plagued by a sweet tooth will understand, is real progress.

Janis and Charles sometimes go out to eat but their main entertainment is going to friends' houses or having them home for a meal. "I love doing that because I enjoy cooking so much," said Janis. "Last week I had a dinner party and we had smoked salmon and prawns on a bed of green salad using different types of lettuce. I made various sauces which people helped themselves to if they wanted. Next we had beef olives with new potatoes, ratatouille, baby corn and broccoli. But I really went over the top with the pudding. I knew one of the blokes likes trifle so I made a kiwi fruit trifle and creme caramel. That was followed by different cheeses."

Sounds wonderful but, needless to say, Janis didn't lose any weight that week. Nor did she lose any sleep over it and quite right. If you can't enjoy a good meal once in a while, what's the point? All you need to do is make up for it by being abstemious for a few days before or afterwards. That's the beauty of changing your eating habits rather than going on a diet, after a while you find you don't want to eat that much very often and so you can afford to "go mad" occasionally.

Being a typical farmer's wife, Janis always has a well-stocked larder full of home-made cakes, bread and biscuits. So temptation is always around.

"We all like our puddings so I still make them but I don't eat anything like the amount I used to. For instance, if you imagine a blackcurrant cheesecake cut into quarters, I will have a third of a quarter. And if I make pancakes they are like crepes, not the thick kind, and I put lemon on and some sweetener or I will have just a dessertspoon of custard and a tablespoon of chocolate pudding. I still want to end a meal with something sweet, even if it is just melon. But I am losing the weight anyway."

Janis has to make a proper meal at lunchtime. "Whereas some women can make do with a snack, when you have a farmer who is coming in at midday, he needs feeding properly. And quite often my daughter or the boys are around at lunchtime as well."

She spends two and a half hours on Mondays, Wednesdays, Fridays and Saturdays delivering milk so felt she was getting enough exercise, especially as Broadbottom is particularly hilly. But the truth is, unless your heart rate is increased substantially, you are not burning off any calories. The milk round may have been keeping her reasonably fit but that's not the same as losing weight. So, about a month into our diet, Janis was persuaded to use the exercise bike she had standing idle in her bedroom.

At first she could only manage five minutes but that is enough to burn off a few calories and get the metabolism speeded up. Gradually she was able to build on that until she was doing half an hour and the more often she does it, the more calories she will burn off, speeding up her metabolism and acquiring a firmer figure into the bargain.

"I feel more alert now, and not so solid. I don't feel it is such an effort to get up the hills as I did before. Nor is it such an effort to get up in the morning. I am pleased with the way my weight has gone down, slowly, because that suits me. There is always something happening in your life, the time of month, a family trauma, or whatever, so I don't think you could lose five or six pounds a week, it wouldn't be natural.

"I came along in the first place because I wanted to start wearing nice clothes again. My wedding dress was only a size 10 and already I'm able to get into clothes I haven't worn for years," she said.

The steady weight loss means Janis went from 13 stone to 10 stone 2 lbs over a period of five months and she is determined to carry on with her new farmer's fare—forever.

FARMER'S FARE

Here is Janis's selection from her weekly menu, if you want to follow her example, choose one from each section—and watch the weight melt like butter in the oven.

Breakfasts (Janis doesn't like to start with anything cooked)
2 oz Muesli or
1 small slice toast
scrape of marmalade, no butter
tea, milk, no sugar

Light Meals
Prawn salad, 2 crispbread, cottage cheese
Ham, two small slices brown bread, salad
Cup of soup, 2 crispbread
2 crispbread and cottage cheese
Homemade coleslaw, low calorie salad cream
*Homemade vegetable soup
Jacket potato and filling (on a cold day)
2 egg omelet, green salad
Banana sandwich
Beans on toast with 1 rasher grilled bacon
Cottage cheese and prawn salad
1 apple, banana or nectarine, whatever is in season
Main Meals
*Chicken stir fry with any vegetables in season. Janis doesn't fry onions, she starts off by sizzling them in apple juice. Serve with boiled rice
Lasagne, salad and broccoli

Steamed fish, new potatoes, peas, sweetcorn
Roast meat, a variety of vegetables in season
gravy but no roast potatoes
Spaghetti Bolognaise
Beef casserole, no potatoes, crispy French loaf
Tuna and pasta bake and salad
Prawn curry with rice

Puds

Small portion baked apples with fruit rather
than pastry
*Bean Pie
Apple pie, cream
Melon
Pancake with lemon and sweetener
Blackcurrant cheesecake
Frozen chocolate gateau
Steamed chocolate pudding and custard

Snacks

Fruit
Yoghurt
low fat Fromage frais on crispbread

Drinks

Wine
Tia Maria and coke is a favourite tipple although Janis doesn't have it
often, just when she craves something sweet
4 glasses water
3 cups fruit tea

The Munchies

JUNE COZENS

Age: 54
Height: 5' 6"
Weight: 12 stone 7 lbs
Target: 10 stone 7 lbs
Weight so far:
10 stone 6 lbs

This has changed my life. That was June's verdict after being hypnotised and following our diet plan for the first month.

June, an interior designer, was desperate to get her figure back, but knew she had the will power of a gnat. That's why being hypnotised appealed to her.

"If I can do it, anybody can," said June. "If you'd said six months ago I'd be able to give up lager and bread, I'd have thought you were mad."

What made June put on weight is a story that hundreds, if not thousands, of women her age will identify with. She was made redundant from her job as the marketing and sales director of a courier company; her four children all married and left home and she had been separated from her husband for about 15 years. So she went from coping with a full-time job and caring for her large family, to having only herself to think about.

Although June set herself up in business making soft furnishings, the pace of life slowed down. Working from home meant she wasn't even getting any exercise going backwards and forwards to an office every day.

"Living on my own, I wasn't eating properly," said June. "My cupboards were bare except for convenience food because I didn't feel the need to cook properly. I just relied mostly on sandwiches and ready-made meals.

"I play in a darts team and all my social life centres around the local pub where I'd think nothing of having nine halves of lager at any one session. Then I'd go home and make myself perhaps four bap sandwiches filled with corned beef or tinned ham. I liked to feel full. But I'd got to the stage where I couldn't see over my stomach and knew I had to do something about it."

Her low point was the early evening. She could go all day without eating but then wanted to gorge—a common failing among people with a weight problem.

"Now I eat less, I am much more active, and I don't even feel as if I'm trying to lose weight."

June's unconscious mind associated eating with comfort.. So hypnosis was the perfect instrument to tackle this deep down problem, and start the process of re-programming her into a healthier approach to living.

Here's how she tackled her programme:

June is the sort of person who is always laughing, especially at herself, in spite of having crippling arthritis.

She says, "The arthritis is not so bad in the summer but in winter I suffer. I sometimes have to take morphine for the pain but I won't let it beat me.

"Before, I was much more sluggish than I am now which I always put down to the arthritis. But as I can now get about so much better, it must have been the fat that was making me tired."

I called June's diet The Munchies because they are the mainstay of her healthy new eating programme. The Munchies came from one of my daughter's friends whom I'd often find rooting around in our fridge. "I've got the munchies," she'd explain. "I hope you don't mind." It became a catch phrase in our house for anyone who suddenly felt hungry and wanted to nibble. That's what June does and she keeps a special airtight container with a ready supply of munchies to keep her going.

Hers are a collection of raw vegetables which June replenishes every two or three days. At first she could hardly believe what she was being asked to do—she'd never eaten raw vegetables before. And as for drinking two litres of water every day, such a change in her drinking habits would have raised a big belly laugh only a short time ago.

Yet here she was, following a one hundred per cent healthy diet - and loving every minute of it. "I am beginning to feel better than I have done for years," she said after only a fortnight. "Not drinking has a lot to do with it, but it's the raw vegetables that most impress me.

"I tuck into them all day, whenever I feel hungry, and I'm still losing weight. I can't be bothered to make fancy dishes so I eat the vegetables plus a jacket potato, some fish or a piece of chicken breast with maybe a steak once a week, and I'm as happy as a sandboy."

Besides following my dietary advice with gusto, June was very enthusiastic about the hypnosis. "I listened to the tape all the time at the beginning but even though I don't listen so much now, what Paul said is always on my mind. It has been a revelation. And it hasn't been hard to follow his advice—this new way of eating comes automatically. He seems to have retrained my mind and my body has responded."

June goes to a yoga class once a week. She also swims once a week but doesn't go fast enough to burn off any fat. Swimming at a slow pace is fine for stamina and toning the muscles, but if you want to lose weight you have to put a spurt on. The secret of burning calories is to get your heart rate up.

June is also a heavy smoker so her metabolism is working under difficult conditions. Having to cope with noxious chemicals, her system obviously isn't going to function efficiently. She'd like to give up smoking but I suggested she gets into a healthier eating pattern first. When she's slimmer, doing lots of exercise and feeling great, she'll have more incentive to give up the dreaded weed.

I put a total ban on the lager, except for high days and holidays and within a very short time June started noticing the difference. So did the regulars at her pub.

"The darts team goes round to different pubs so there are a lot of people who are amazed when they see me. Darts girls scream a lot and they have been letting out some mega screams at my new figure. Which is very satisfying.

"But I haven't given up drinking altogether. Now I'm slimmer, I allow myself a couple of Pils at the end of the evening- because I think it has less sugar than draught."

June has also managed to cut down on the number of cups of coffee and tea she drinks in a day because she has taken on board the fact that caffeine debilitates the metabolism. "If someone comes I might make a brew but I don't necessarily have one," she said. "I have a glass of water instead. It is more difficult to drink cold water in the winter so I've switched to things like hot Bovril, Marmite or lemon and ginger, so I still get the liquid."

June used to keep bread in her freezer so there were always baps on tap but now she has only the odd crispbread. Not that bread is a no-go area for people who want to lose weight. But because June was so addicted to it, I thought it was probably a good idea for her to give it up, at least for a while.

The great advantage of having a ready-made supply of munchies is you have something instant to eat. As every dieter knows, you can chomp your way through 300 calories just waiting for something "sensible" to cook. Pour dressing over your munchies or have a dip ready - but don't overdose on the dips because calories can creep up on you unawares that way. Add munchies to a couple of crispbreads and cottage cheese, follow that plateful with an apple, orange or other fruit - and you will be extremely well fed.

Since June can't be bothered to count calories her diet diary looks pretty repetitive, the same old thing every day. But it suits her and that's all that matters. People who live on their own tend to stick to a few basic dishes week in week out, it's only the odd day when they feel like treating themselves or when they have people coming they make something a bit different. And if you're on a diet, the most important thing is to eat in a way that is going to give you the least hassle. Most of us like to have something we can dive into quickly which is why I predict The Munchies will be one of the most popular "diets" of the series.

"I'm not bored with it," she says. "So long as I have my bowl of vegetables I can be full in two ticks. My mother who is 90 is often over here and my family come at weekends with my grandchildren and I give them all the munchies for a snack and they love it.

"For main meals I cook basic things like liver and onions and I like steak done in onions. I also do fish in milk, I think it's potty to dress fish up with fancy sauces when it tastes perfectly good grilled or poached. I don't use the frying pan any more, I threw that out after our first meeting when you talked about how bad for you fried food is.

"One of my neighbours goes fishing so I get fresh trout and mackerel from him quite a lot. And I buy haddock. I also eat a lot of sardines and pilchards now. I've started to have them for breakfast on toast."

June takes cod liver oil for her arthritis, and she has been told by her doctor to keep off citrus fruits. Calves' liver, sardines, brown rice, beans and poultry are all items to include in her weekly diet which may help to alleviate the symptoms.

"After the first month on this new healthy eating plan my skin and hair started to look and feel much better but since my arthritis got really bad, it's all gone to cock. God knows, though, what I would have looked like if I had been eating and drinking like I used to."

When June came to our weigh-ins she'd be showing off the jeans she hadn't worn for years, or pulling them out from her waist to see how baggy they were getting. She was prouder of her progress than any of our other dieters. Even when she went on holiday to Tunisia with a friend, she came back having lost weight.

"When I went to Blackpool with four friends for the weekend I was amazed at how two of them who are only in their early forties, had to go to sleep in the afternoons," said this transformed new woman. "The best thing this diet has done for me is rejuvenation. I'm not sluggish any more."

THE MUNCHIES
This is what June's healthy eating programme consists of:

Daily: Half a pint of semi-skimmed milk for drinks or cereals

Breakfasts
    1 slice wholemeal toast, scrape margarine plus yeast extract
    Sardines on toast
    Pilchards on toast
    All Bran or muesli
    Fruit juice and/or tea

Light meals
    Munchies:
    a mixture of whatever vegetables are available like
    cauliflower, red and green pepper, spring onions,
    cucumber, celery, mushrooms (but only added as she is
    about to eat her munchies because they sweat), courgettes,
    apple, parsley, lettuce, water cress—plus French dressing

Or one of the following:
1 tablespoon cottage cheese and 1 or 2 crispbreads
Sardines on toast
Sandwich with salad and ham, cooked chicken or turkey
Smoked mackerel with one bap
Scrambled egg on toast

Main meals

Soup to start. June is particularly fond of clear
Chinese soups. Followed by one of these:
100g grilled steak with two cooked vegetables
Grilled pork or lamb chop with at least two cooked vegetables
*Speedy Plaice with Leeks and Potato
1 jacket potato with 1 oz butter, baked beans
Grilled bacon and tomatoes
*Liver and Bacon in tomato sauce
*Fish Tikka
Lean cuisines with liver or beef and dumplings
Ready made spaghetti bolognaise with bowl munchies
Wholemeal pasta with lean mince, onions, carrots, celery
Rabbit with barley, carrots and onions
Grilled haddock, dotted with sunflower margarine
Low cal yoghurt
Fresh fruit or fruit salad

Drinks

Mixed fruit juice
tomato juice
2 cups coffee a day
2 cups of tea
1-2 litres water

Snacks

Fresh fruit
Crispbread with low fat soft cheese
Bowl of munchies

Treats
>   Pils lager
>   Chinese meal

June's family visit her constantly she so she has a broad range of recipes she uses as well as making sure she is eating the right things to help relieve her arthritis. She is also very fond of Chinese food so has chosen some of those from our recipe section.

Chinese wrapped chicken
Sweet and sour drumsticks
Seafish Creole
Prawn Madras
Pork with leeks and lentils
Liver and paprika
Autumn vegetable casserole
Mackerel pate
Smoked haddock pate
Captain's fish bake
Mince, leek and potato bake
Stir fry with orange and chilli
Cottage pie
Lentils and pasta
Kipper stir fry
Herring kebabs

Brown Owl's Diet

ANNE JONES

Age: 43
Height: 5' 8"
Weight: 11 stone 7 lbs
Target: 10 stone 7 lbs
Weight so far: 10 stone 2 lbs

Anne is a dinner lady, married with four children aged 24, 22, 18 and 6. She is also leader of the village's brownies—their Brown Owl.

Although she wasn't grossly overweight, Anne was very keen to get slimmer and was gratified by her husband's compliments as soon as the difference became obvious.

She admitted she had a weakness—for cups of tea. "Sometimes as many as 10 a day, with biscuits," she said.

Her dinner lady duties also led her into temptation. "When I'm working at school I may have a muffin with corned beef and tomato for lunch," said Anne. Well, that isn't too bad, except corned beef does contain quite a bit of fat—there are just over 200 calories in 100 grams (about 3 ounces). Anne's lunch would probably add up to between 400-500 calories. Which doesn't leave much for the rest of the day.

But, anyway, she spoilt her otherwise fairly healthy-sounding lunch by admitting, "And I can't resist their lovely puds." Having chocolate eclairs and jam doughnuts under your nose would tax the will power of a saint, and Anne regularly gave in to temptation.

Like all overweight people, Anne needed to re-programme her eating habits. So, with the help of the Hypno Slim tape, she set about finding a new approach to food.

Here's how she did it: At first Anne didn't think she'd be able to give

29

up the tea but when she understood how poisonous it is (just picture what comes out of your tea pot when you clean it...) she made up her mind to give it a really good try.

And she surprised herself. Within six weeks Anne was drinking the required amount of water, two litres, and not missing her cups of tea as much as she thought she would. It has to be said this was achieved mostly during the school holidays and as soon as the term started again Anne went back to her tea drinking habit—and put on a few pounds.

Even though she didn't resume munching biscuits, the tea was enough to stop her metabolism in its tracks. This can happen and it's the same with coffee for some people. The more caffeine they drink the less efficient their system becomes.

The daily diary, which every dieter ought to keep up religiously but few do, was a must. It let us see where she was going wrong. And hey presto, the discipline of keeping the diary concentrated Anne's mind on what she was eating.

When you don't keep a record, you can kid yourself. But a food intake diary acts like a brake on your appetite.

And Anne's family tries to help. "My youngest son, Adam, refuses to give me any of his crisps or toffees now because he knows I'm trying to lose weight. And I have stopped buying packets of biscuits—which no one seems to have noticed. If Adam wants something sweet I just buy him a Kit Kat or something similar so there is nothing around to tempt me."

Anne suffers from an iron deficiency so we recommended she include liver at least once or preferably twice a week in her diet and to add red kidney beans to some of her other meals.

"I don't have much will power so for me hypnosis was a very welcome aid," she said. "I've tried Paul's exercise with the voice, the one that is telling me it is OK to indulge when I want something sweet, by making it sound like Mickey Mouse, but it doesn't always work.

"One day I ate everything I could get hold of in the house, two cakes and a trifle!" Another day she bought a packet of Penguin biscuits, thought she'd just have one and ended up eating four! Needless to say, Anne didn't lose any weight that week.

In fact, she didn't lose any for three weeks sometimes, which can be depressing but, besides the fact that sometimes she was over-eating, Anne had to come to terms with the fact that the body does adjust to a new level of calorie intake. And it gets harder to lose weight the less you have to lose.

Never mind, the beauty of pacing yourself to reach a long-term goal is that you can afford to fall by the wayside occasionally. We are all human and it would be a miracle if you could suddenly change to a healthy, non-fattening diet after years of indulging in bad habits

What we are out to prove with the help of hypnosis is that you can learn new ways of eating but, as Paul says, you have to have patience and be persistent. One of the reasons fast diets don't work is that as soon as you come off them, having achieved some sort of goal, you go right back to eating the way you did before. And you end up on the weight-gain-weight-loss merry-go-round. Except it isn't so merry.

One unfortunate side effect which Anne found on her diet was she suddenly developed really bad eczema. It started first just as two spots on her arms and then spread all over her body. The doctor gave her special cream and she changed her washing powder and put everything into the washing machine, including the bed linen, but still she was suffering very badly.

Obviously one area to look at was her diet and, because she had started to eat low-fat yoghurt and cottage cheese as part of her new regime, they were considered possible suspects. And sure enough, when she stopped eating them, the eczema went away.

It is a salutary lesson. Finding out what foods you are allergic to can often be painstaking and in Anne's case she suffered a lot of discomfort until the culprits were established. So even if it is a chore, keeping a diet diary can pay worthwhile dividends.

Anne went on her first holiday abroad in the middle of our experiment but did not put on any weight. And she was thrilled with her slimmer shape. "I had to buy a new swimming costume because my old one kept slipping off my shoulders," she said. "That made me feel very good. I did a bit of swimming but the water was very cold so didn't do a lot. I don't take any exercise normally, I just don't have the time."

That is what a lot of busy people say. Anne has 18 brownies to cater for in the community centre and she does walk up and down to the school

31

four times a day. Besides which, she has her husband and four children to look after so she is kept on the move all the time.

"I hardly ever sit down so I don't know where I'd find an hour in the day to do proper exercises," she said.

It is a question of discipline and allotting time to yourself, something women are not brilliant at. But at least in other ways Anne has changed her life considerably and I am still hoping that one day she will stop long enough to give her body a healthy workout.

"I feel much better since I started the eating programme which I think has a lot to do with the raw and extra green vegetables I am eating. I don't have as many potatoes and also think about what to eat to counteract the lack of iron. Now I have liver twice a week I don't feel as tired as I used to."

She confessed to a chocolate binge once our weekly weigh-ins had stopped but says: "I didn't enjoy it and I can't see myself ever doing it again. I was like a kid who had been let loose but now my sweet tooth seems to have gone.

"The best thing of all about the hypnosis and learning to eat properly is being able to get into clothes I haven't worn for years - without having to resort to safety pins!"

BROWN OWL'S DIET

Breakfasts
2 slices white toast
low fat spread
1 mug tea, semi skimmed milk, sweetener

Light meals
sandwiches of every description with salad
raw vegetables with dips
jacket potato with cottage cheese
sardines on toast
vegetable soup and bap
fresh fruit

Main meals

*Vegetable bake
*Italian liver
*Fisherman's pie
Tuna Pasta bake
Lasagne
Calves liver, onions, mashed potatoes and green vegetables
*Pork and pineapple stir fry
*Sweet and Sour drumsticks
Spaghetti Bolognaise
Sugar free jelly
Sugar free Angel Delight

Snacks

Marmite on toast
Fresh fruit

Treats

Chocolate eclairs
Milky bars

The Wok Pot

ANDREW FAITHFUL	PAULINE FAITHFUL
Age: 35	Age: 34
Height: 6' 1"	Height: 5' 5"
Weight: 18 stone 10lbs	Weight: 14 stone 4lbs
Target: 14 stone 7 lb	Target: 10 stone 7lbs
Weight so far:	Weight so far:
16 stone 7 lbs	12 stone 7 lbs

Andrew is a policeman and Pauline looks after their two children, Laura aged three and Thomas, two. She was her target weight when they married five years ago but put on the pounds when she became pregnant with Laura. She went up to 12 stones. Eight months later, before she'd had time to lose the first lot of extra weight, she became pregnant again. During her second pregnancy Pauline shot up to 14 stone.

Because she takes care of her appearance, has lovely glossy hair and trim ankles, Pauline doesn't appear to be as big as she is—a problem many women share. Their weight is so well disguised they don't realise they're getting fat. Or at least they find it easy to ignore.

We've heard of husbands getting sympathy pains during a wife's pregnancy but in Andrew's case it was his weight which matched Pauline's. By the time she started to worry about her weight he, too, was beginning to look like a seriously big bobby.

Most of his flab was around his chest and stomach which spells danger—medical experts have proved, when your excess fat makes you the shape of a plump pigeon, you are more prone to heart attacks. Women are mostly spared that since their weight usually settles on the hips and thighs.

Both Andrew and Pauline had tried dieting before with no success and they both have weaknesses. Pauline's is nibbling at crisps and biscuits and Andrew couldn't resist a visit to the chippy when he was on night duty. His other weakness will be familiar to many parents: he finished up what the children left on their plates.

Both found the hypnosis worked right from the start. "My mother-in-law looked after the children while we were being hypnotised and she'd made them some chips," said Andrew. "Yet when I went to pick them up I didn't want any! Amazing!"

During the first week Pauline reported the same sort of reaction. "Even when we took the children out and I bought them a cake, I only had a taste and didn't want any more. Normally I would have had a piece of chocolate cake all to myself."

Both Andrew's and Pauline's unconscious minds associated eating pleasure with the wrong kinds of food. It's possible to eat plenty of delicious things and stay healthy and slim—as long as they're the *right* things. But this message had not reached their unconscious minds until they began the Hypno Slim programme.

Here's how they arrested their bad habits:

Andrew is luckier than Pauline because he has a gym at the police station where he's been able to go on the exercise bike or rowing machine for 25 minutes every day. He reckons he cycles for nine miles and probably works off a few hundred calories doing that.

Exercise, of course, not only burns fat, it also helps to speed up your metabolism so he is a double winner.

They have an exercise bike at home with the kind of moving handlebars that make you exercise your upper half as well but Pauline can't do it while she's alone with the children because they poke their fingers through the spokes. (There are new ones which don't have spokes so are much safer when you have small children around but they are expensive. Look in the local paper small ads section for good second-hand buys.)

"Even when Andrew is there to look after the children, almost as soon as I disappear to our bedroom to start pedalling they shout, 'Where's Mummy?'" she said.

That's something Pauline—and every mother of young children has to be strong about—the need to insist on ME time. Children tend to know when Mum wants to be alone and always kick up a fuss if they can possibly stop her. But if she insists on half an hour alone, they'll survive. It's not being selfish to allow ME time. In the long run it's being sensible.

Pauline did manage to squeeze a small space of time for herself - 12 minutes to be exact. She bought the Y Plan exercise video which has been put together by the YWCA and is one of the best exercise tapes, in my opinion. Also, because it is short, you can get down to doing it with less hassle.

"It is split into 4 levels and I am just doing level 1 because it's years since I did any exercise," said Pauline. "At first I thought the actual exercises were quite easy until I realised I wasn't doing them as I should. As I started to take more notice, I got into the right positions and could feel more pull. The exercises are really well-organised and there is a cooling down period to finish off.

"The second set are aerobics and I get really puffed out by the end of it. They have made me feel I might quite enjoy going to an aerobics class."

Pauline had a bad bout of bronchitis at the beginning of the programme so she had another excuse for not sticking to her diet as rigidly as she might.

On the other hand, two stones is not bad going by anyone's reckoning and, sensibly, Pauline is happy to take her time. If she loses another two stones by the summer she will reach her target.

As I keep saying, it's the fast fad diets which don't work. Adjusting your eating pattern takes longer but lasts longer, too.

What the Faithfuls did do—faithfully—was weigh all their food. And it came as a shock to realise just how much more they had been cooking of late. Increasing the amount of food you prepare is another way weight creeps on without you noticing.

"I remember when we were first married we used to make a meal then freeze some of it, but gradually we began to eat everything," said Andrew. "Obviously that was part of the problem."

Another problem they had was eating too late at night. Often they'd wait until the children were in bed but that could mean it was 9pm before they had their main meal of the day - the worst possible time. Just when the metabolism is slowing down preparing the body for sleep.

Following my advice, they swopped their main meal to midday whenever possible and just had a light meal in the evening with the children. Admittedly, for a shift worker, this is sometimes difficult but, equally, when Andrew starts at three in the afternoon, it fits into his work schedule perfectly.

Pauline and Andrew's biggest initial success was to cut out nibbling in between meals. And that, they say, was thanks to Paul.

"I feel the hypnotism works in everyday life, too," said Pauline. "If something gets you down, it's easier, with the advice you get from Paul, to step sideways mentally and look at things differently.

"I like his idea of imagining something that makes you happy or a place you would like to be because it does have a calming effect. It is as easy to make yourself smile as it is to make yourself unhappy by thinking about something sad.

"The words Paul uses encourage you to eat more healthily. He says you will eat only as much as your body wants, if you listen to your body, you won't over-eat."

And Andrew added, "I can make chips for the children now and not want any."

Andrew is the cook in the family. He loves it, and tends to make up his own recipes as he goes along, forever experimenting. He is a great enthusiast of the wok way of cooking, throwing vegetables, spices and herbs into the mixture as the fancy takes him. In the north, a previous generation used to rely on the stewpot for their filling dinners. Andrew's wok is the modern-day healthy equivalent, which is why I christened their diet The Wokpot, because it's a mixture of both.

The only thing you have to make sure of is you don't use too much oil. In fact you can substitute carrot, tomato, orange or apple juice or stock for oil and still get fantastic results. But you mustn't fall into the trap the Faithfuls fell into, and gradually make too much. It's a hazard of wok cooking because it is so easy to throw more and more into a whacking great wok. The fact it tastes so delicious doesn't help either!

Andrew has had an allotment for two years and grows lots of their own vegetables including onions, spinach, broccoli, beans and potatoes. They also have a small bay tree and some red and green chillies growing on their kitchen window. Andrew is also a canny shopper. He uses Basmati rice he buys from a local Indian warehouse and once bought an enormous bag of lentils, weighing five kilos, for just £1.30.

About eight years ago Pauline became intolerant of animal fats. "I used to get welts and my skin started to burn, it was an itchy sensation that was very unpleasant," she said. "I used to eat a lot of cheese and I still like it and we eat it occasionally but nothing on the scale I used to. And I only ever have skimmed milk."

We decided right at the beginning that Pauline probably needed more vitamins and besides changing her diet she also opted for a multi-vitamin containing extra calcium and iron. Now she proudly shows off beautiful long finger nails which she hasn't had since her first baby was born.

Since she seemed to be plagued with throat and chest infections vitamin A was obviously called for and one of the snacks she has now developed a taste for is garlic and chives pitta bread spread with Marmite.

"Yeast extract was something I never fancied before but I'm getting to like it," said Pauline. Spinach, sweet potatoes, spring greens and eggs are also good sources of vitamin A, though not for Pauline because she can't eat eggs.

They are almost, though not quite, vegetarians so Pauline doesn't ever eat liver which is a pity because it is another valuable source of the essential vitamins she needs. It's just as well, then, that Andrew chucks lentils into many of the dishes he concocts because they are rich in iron and phosphorus as well as the B vitamins.

Neither Andrew nor Pauline could entertain a fast day or even a vegetable only day but when they were being good they were very, very good. Their scrupulous weighing of everything meant they could keep track of what was going into the wok.

And Pauline, very sensibly, is happy for her weight loss programme to take a long time. "I couldn't lose a stone a month, it just wouldn't be realistic. I want to lose this weight and keep it off forever. Also dieting would just make me depressed. We still go to the takeaway and I'm sure if we didn't do that we would lose more quickly but I'm not bothered. I feel alright and I am enjoying doing it."

Andrew was better at drinking the quota of water. Some days Pauline only managed one glass but, as she points out, that's a 100 per cent improvement on what she drank before. And she admits, "Often I would start drinking more on a Monday and by the weigh-in on Wednesday I'd either have lost another pound or at least stayed the same and I'm sure it was the extra water that helped. I can see I'm going to have to do a lot more work on that to turn it into a habit."

The greatest difference Pauline has noticed since she started our diet is that she doesn't feel so tired. "Before we started I would, say, go to clean the bathroom and only manage the sink and toilet. I couldn't do the shower cubicle, I'd have to go and have a drink and sit down so it would take me two days to clean the bathroom properly.

Now I can start at the top of the house and work my way down, cleaning the three bedrooms and the bathroom. And that means cleaning windows, dusting, vacuuming, doing it really well."

I have a feeling the Faithfuls will make progress slowly—but they'll get there in the end.

THE WOKPOT
Breakfasts:

> Pauline - Cereal or
> > Toast with no butter, scrape of marmalade
> > Coffee with milk, no sugar
> Andrew - 2 oz Cornflakes, porridge with 2 oz dried fruit,
> > Weetabix, or fruit 'n fibre
> > On high days and holidays Andrew indulges in
> > Grilled sausage, bacon, tomato and egg and Pauline
> > has grilled tomato and mushrooms on
> > wholemeal bread

Light meals

> Tuna salad
> Tuna fish with sauce and pasta
> Sandwiches with Edam cheese and salad, no butter but
> spiced with low fat Thousand Island Dressing, mustard or
> vinaigrette dressing
> Jacket potato with cottage cheese or beans
> Mushroom soup
> Scrambled eggs on toast (Andrew)
> Cheese on toast (Pauline)
> Grilled mackerel
> Fresh fruit

Main meals

Wok mix:
*Diced chicken or turkey with a variety of vegetables and pulses plus garlic, soy sauce, cumin seeds and lemon juice served with pasta or rice

Chicken breast rubbed with garlic and roasted and served with a selection of vegetables or baked potato

Mince fried in own fat, onions and garlic, tin tomatoes, celery, aubergines and spiced with oregano, served with pasta or baked potato

Turkey roast in oven with tikka paste and yoghurt, herbs and Bhuna paste served with rice

Spaghetti Bolonaise

Coq au Vin, boiled potatoes

Pumpkin Soup with star-shaped pasta

Snacks

Ryvita with cheese

Handful of raisins

Marmite on pitta bread

Fruit

Treats

Ice cream

Wine, both red and white

Irish coffee with aerosol cream and sweeteners

Drinks

Andrew 6-8 cups of tea and coffee daily

Pauline 5-6 decaf coffees

Andre 1 litre Water and Pauline 1 glass

Andrew loves his wok so his favourite recipes are nearly all ones you can cook just by throwing in whatever takes your fancy: a mixture of meat or fish and vegetables then stir-frying them for 6-10 minutes or until the vegetables are tender.

Sweet Temptations

BRENDA LEE	DAVID LEE
Age: 45	Age: 46
Height: 5' 4"	Height: 5' 8"
Weight: 11 stone 5 lbs	Weight: 14 stone
Target: 9 stone 7 lbs	Target: 12 stone
Weight so far:	Weight so far:
10 stone 2 lbs	12 stone 12 lbs

B renda Lee has two newspaper shops so she and David are surrounded by sweets, crisps, ices, chocolate and sugary soft drinks. The temptations for them are terrible.

On top of that, their day starts earlier than most people's. There is a dog to walk and the morning papers to be delivered. They have a cup of tea at quarter to five in the morning and a proper, often cooked, breakfast at 8.30.

After that Brenda doesn't have much time to prepare elaborate meals because she is busy serving in the shop all day. She only closes for an hour at lunchtime when she needs a nap after that early start so shopping and cooking have to be pared down to the bare minimum.

In the evening she usually starts dinner at six so by the time David, who had to give up his job as a postman because of arthritis in the knees, is ready to eat at seven, there is a substantial supper ready. These need to be fairly easy to make because she has to dart between the kitchen and the shop which is still open.

Another problem for them is David's sweet tooth. How to satisfy him and still lose weight? That was, at the beginning, Brenda's biggest worry.

She had already managed to lose some weight before we started, for their son's wedding, but she felt she still had a long way to go. "I'm very interested in trying hypnosis," she said. "I feel as if I have gone as far as I can under my own steam."

David thought doing the diet together would make it easier for them both and was impressed with the way the hypnosis made him rethink what he was putting into his mouth. "I am forever picking at bars of chocolate," he admitted.

Here's their good news story:

David found that after the hypnosis he stopped picking. He says, "Occasionally I'll get a yearning for something sweet. Once I had seven small eccles cakes at once but it didn't seem to make any difference to my weight. I still managed to lose that week.

"I could never pick at rabbit food, salads and such. And tea without sugar leaves a horrible taste in your mouth. But I have now managed to cut it down to just a quarter of a teaspoonful. If you had told me a few months ago I would stop nibbling at chocolate bars and biscuits, I'd never have believed it."

David was thrilled when he could wear a pair of trousers he had not worn for years and Brenda could not convince a friend she wasn't starving herself to get slim. "I'm not saying it's been easy, but I have been eating quite a lot. Or at least quite a lot considering I am supposed to be dieting."

Unlike David who managed to get away with not being "good" on the odd occasion, Brenda found when she wasn't "good" the scales immediately revealed all. It's not fair! How often have you heard about people who lose weight easily compared to others who try just as hard and it take forever to lose that fat? We're all built differently and you just have to be patient with yourself.

Brenda and David went to Spain for a week's holiday in the middle of our diet programme and although they had a bit more to drink than usual, they were careful about what they ate. But they didn't let dieting come between them and having a good time—I'm glad to say.

"David had the puddings at our hotel but I stuck to fruit and enjoyed that very much," said Brenda. "We weren't going to go on holiday and be miserable."

I would have been disappointed with them if they had done anything else. To pay all that money for a holiday abroad and then spend your mealtimes worrying about how many calories you are eating would be murder. Part of the fun of holidays is eating foreign food and not having to cook it, shop for it, or clean up afterwards. Calorie counting would put a real dampener on that.

Anyway, when they returned Brenda and David had hardly put on any weight, just a pound each. It just goes to show that once the metabolism is working well, you can afford to relax sometimes without any terrible consequences. Diets where you are restricted even at times when you are supposed to be celebrating fail in the end because you end up feeling miserable and resentful. You think, 'What's life about?'

The Lees also had family celebrations like a 21st birthday party and meeting up with friends for a night out when they didn't want to be party poopers, so my advice was: forget dieting. What you do on those occasions is, instead of having seconds of the glorious puds on offer, fill up on food from the "good" list. It isn't easy and if you do give in to temptation, you can always make up for it by being extra frugal the next day.

Brenda definitely finds dieting harder than David: when she's hungry she aches and has to have something. And funnily enough, she can't have an apple, she insists they make her more hungry. But she loves pomegranates so when they are in season treats herself to a between-meals snack with one of those. Or she chooses a low calorie soup with, perhaps, a couple of crispbreads—instead of a bag of crisps or a chocolate bar, which is what she automatically ate before.

It really isn't a good idea to let yourself get to the stage where your hunger is taking over. Much better to give your stomach something to gnaw on then you can ignore it and get on with your life. Some nutritionists argue it is better to eat fruit on an empty stomach and I certainly feel full up after I've eaten an apple, pear or banana. Brenda sounds unlucky but for most of us it is much better not to have fruit as a desert and save it up instead for those times when you feel starving.

It is often the cup of tea or coffee that David and Brenda drink which lures them into having a biscuit to go with it and although I suggested they forget those beverages and stick to water, the suggestion didn't meet with much enthusiasm. David only drinks about one pint of water although he has switched to low or no cal soft drinks in place of the sugar-rich ones. Brenda reckons she probably gets through two pints of water a day but that is nowhere near the two litres which everyone needs to drink.

A few years ago if someone had tried to persuade me to drink two litres of water a day, I would have thought it was impossible. Yet now I some-times drink even more and think nothing of it. When you go into the kitchen to make a cup of tea, while you're waiting for the kettle to boil, more often than not you reach for the biscuit tin. Right? But if you have a bottle of water beside you, there is no temptation to go wandering in the direction of the chocolate digestives.

Brenda has bottles of water in her fridge in the shop so she can help herself as often as she likes. She is trying, but it still feels like a penance, she doesn't enjoy it.

Both Brenda and David, for different reasons, find it almost impossible to exercise. Brenda is stuck behind the counter every day, although she was toying with the idea of getting an exercise bicycle. "I could put it in the passage between the shop and the house and cycle when we have no customers," she said. It would make sense because although losing fat is important, it is also important to firm up your muscles so you get a good figure.

David can't do any exercise because of his arthritis and it is difficult for him to walk, never mind try jogging, cycling or aerobics. Since he started our diet, however, he has found himself much more mobile. He went up a ladder for the first time since he couldn't remember when, which was a small but significant achievement.

Like a lot of people who lead busy lives, even after a lot of discussion, they couldn't see where they would find room for exercise. I do sympa-thise. Unless you are incredibly keen on keeping fit or there is something local you feel like joining, there really is no incentive to turn out on a cold winter's night. It's hard to convince anyone that once you've done some strenuous exercises, you will actually feel less tired and more cheerful.

You can see the expression on people's faces when you try to explain it to them: pull the other one, it says. Most people prefer to relax with a glass of wine or beer in front of the television.

David has an unusual way of unwinding: he has become an expert at dry stone walling. It is a hobby which is absorbing and incredibly popular in the area—even young children are keen and groups of twenty or more learn how to do it when the weather is fine.

Brenda plays darts on Tuesday evenings—when she is tempted by the sandwiches laid on by the pub. But her favourite hobby is icing cakes.

At the time of our experiment, she was also in the middle of papering a wall, so when you talk to her about taking time off to do some strenuous exercise, you can understand why she gives you an old fashioned look! Still, I was there to help her lose weight and my advice was: give up the darts, the cake icing or the home improvement and take up something that gets the old ticker pounding.

David, too, could do vigorous exercises involving the top half of his body, lifting weights and so on which would get his heart racing. Even 10 minutes a day would make all the difference.

Fish oil helps to relieve arthritis and David has been taking cod liver oil tablets for a year although he can't bring himself to swallow the oil straight which is supposed to be so much more effective. I suggested he include as many meals as possible with oily fish such as kippers, sardines, herrings, trout and mackerel which may, in the long term, help to ease his joints. Unfortunately, I suspect it is a diet he should have started many years ago. We'll see.

Brenda and David eat quite a lot of white fish and very little red meat so other than the sweet things and not enough water, their diet was already pretty healthy.

"We listen to our hypnosis tape regularly, it helps us to focus on healthy eating," said Brenda. "At the beginning we used to have it on nearly every day but now we only listen about once a week. Often it sends us to sleep, which isn't surprising since we're both so tired all the time, but the message is obviously getting through."

SWEET TEMPTATIONS

Breakfasts

Special K 1oz (Brenda) 2oz (David) plus same amount of Bran Flakes

David will have half a spoon of sugar in his tea and 1 slice toast with light extra Flora

Grilled bacon and egg cooked in juice from bacon

Poached egg on toast

Scrambled egg on toast

1 or 2 boiled eggs and toast

Sundays: grilled bacon, low fat sausages, mushrooms, grilled tomato and toast

Light Meals

Jacket potato with coleslaw or baked beans
Tin of wholewheat spaghetti
Tuna in mayonnaise sauce with sweet corn on a jacket potato
Low cal soup and wholemeal sandwiches with salad and ham or chicken
Scrambled eggs on toast
Boneless kippers in a bag
*Californian pineapple and ham salad
Fish fingers with
*Apple and nut salad with wholemeal bread
Sardines on toast
Grilled mackerel with green salad
Fresh fruit
Low fat yoghurts

Main meals

Liver and onions, string beans, peas, one or two boiled potatoes
Roast chicken with white sauce spiced with mustard, new potatoes, beans, onions
White fish poached in milk and the milk made into a cheese sauce to pour over cauliflower
Ready-cooked Ocean Pie, spinach and carrots
*Pasta salad
*Souffle potato bake
Grilled plaice/cod in sauce
*Lamb casserole, broccoli and cauliflower
Low fat ice cream
Sugar free jelly with fresh fruit

Snacks

Fruit
Low calorie chocolate bar
Coffee and half-fat biscuit or digestive
Tea with low-fat cheese spread on crispbread or wholemeal bread

Treats

Chinese meal
Cheesecake

Bottle of wine

Because Brenda has to work such long hours she relies on recipes that are easy to prepare or she can make in advance. As well as watching what they eat from the calorie point of view, Brenda also tries to include meals which may help to alleviate David's arthritis. Here are some of her choices—you will find them in the back of the book. She also, occasionally, wants to indulge David's sweet tooth.

Smoked haddock pate
Kidneys Turbigo
Potato and smoked mackerel salad
Chive and mackerel pate
Roquefort souffle potatoes
Speedy plaice withleeks and potato
Lamb and leek potato bake
Kipper stir fry
Oaty chicken
Captain's fish bake
Fish tikka
Lemon cheesecake
Chocolate mousse

HYPNO SLIM

Nutrition Guide

GET WISE TO THE FACTS ABOUT FOOD

Y ou need to become your own detective-cum-doctor and get to
know as much as you can about what your body needs and likes.
There is plenty to learn! But for the purposes of losing weight
there are just a few fairly basic facts you should take on board before you
start. By the time you reach your target weight, you will be surprised at
how much knowledge of nutrition you have picked up. After that you
will want to stick to a healthy diet. In fact, I wouldn't mind betting you'll
wonder why you overloaded your body before with so much stuff that
was doing it such a lot of harm.

Calories

A calorie is an internationally recognised way of measuring food into
tiny units of energy (really they ought to be called kilocalories which is
one thousand calories). One calorie is equal to the amount of energy or
heat needed to raise the temperature of one gram of water one degree
centigrade. We need energy to maintain our body temperature at 98.6
degrees Fahrenheit even when we are doing nothing and calories, me-
tabolised by the body, provide us with the fuel to breathe, walk, push a
pen, vacuum or boogie the night away. They are the same "size" whether
they come from fat, protein or carbohydrate—although obviously 500
calories of butter would have a different effect on the torso from 500
calories of cabbage. If you eat more calories than you burn up, the body
stores the excess away as fat, ready for tomorrow in case it gets no fuel at
all. It's a very clever and sensitive machine the body, so you should treat
it with respect.

Counting calories is a favourite pastime of dieters and, in my opinion,
totally useless. Most people who do it religiously end up sooner or later
back where they started—if not weighing even more than before. My
mother lost stones through weighing every morsel that passed her lips all

51

day every day. But five years later, I'm afraid, once she'd given up that tedious nonsense, she was back to her old plump self.

Sure, you should read labels carefully but don't become a calorie-counting slave. None of our Broadbottom dieters did and they all lost the weight they wanted. Some of them even lost more. Also—and this is important—they enjoyed themselves because they didn't feel they were being punished.

Carbohydrates

A carbohydrate is a complex molecule composed of carbon, oxygen and hydrogen and is produced by plants. Carbohydrates are an important source of energy, each gram providing approximately four calories. Carbohydrates are broken down by the body into glucose and any excess is stored in the liver and muscles in the form of glycogen. An abnormal amount of excess carbohydrates—i.e. the realm fat people slide into—is converted into fat.

Without getting too technical about it, the speed with which carbohydrates effect the glycaemic level of your blood determines whether they are "good" or "bad". Glycaemia is the level of glucose in your blood stream which is constantly kept stable by the pancreas secreting insulin.

"Bad" carbohydrates cause a large rise in blood glucose whereas "good" ones don't. I'm only telling you this to illustrate how complicated our digestive system is and any simplistic solution to losing weight is bound, therefore, to be suspect.

Basically there are two kinds of carbohydrates, sugar and starch. Starches are complex carbohydrates: unrefined like wholewheat bread, brown rice and pasta, pulses, potatoes and root vegetables, or refined—the kind you get in cakes, biscuits and cereals. Starches are broken down by the body to be released into energy at a slow and steady rate. Sugars, on the other hand, are fast kick-starters but not as satisfying because they don't have the bulk of complex starches.

Contrary to popular myth, carbohydrates are an essential part of a slimmer's diet because they fill you up, they are awash with vitamins and nutrients and they are our main source of energy.

As a general rule, I'd say the less carbohydrates are mucked about with, the better they are going to be for you because chemical processing raises their glycaemic impact, making it harder for the system to change them into useful fuel. Instead, it stores what it can't handle as superfluous fat.

Choose: wholemeal or rye bread, wholewheat pasta, brown rice, pulses such as lentils, chick peas, dried beans and peas, leeks, turnips, green vegetables, fresh or stewed fruit.

Avoid: beer, spirits, white bread, white rice, refined sugar, beetroot, instant potato, dried fruit, jam, honey, popcorn, sugared cereals and chocolate bars.

Cheese

Delicious though it is, cheese contains a lot of fat and so, for the purposes of dieting, it is virtually a no-go area. Even cottage cheese has its pitfalls and you have to make sure you read the labels carefully because some brands contain sugar. You also have to make sure you drain off the liquid to avoid the whey which contains lactose, a carbohydrate.

If you really like a good cheese, treat yourself to a portion at the end of every month when you have lost enough weight to feel you deserve a relaxation of the rules. Always buy a low-fat cheese for sandwiches because, by the time you have added tomato and lettuce (which you will do, now, won't you?) no one will notice the difference. And if you want to make a cheese sauce, choose the strongest flavour then you will need to use less.

Chocolate

When you eat chocolate, for whatever reason—often just because it's there but usually because you feel hungry, need a pick-me-up, are depressed or succumbing to a habit—you are doing yourself and your body a great disservice. Sugary snacks are devoid of any nutrients, all they contain is loads of calories, and you are forcing your body to use up its vital stock of vitamins and minerals in order to digest these refined carbohydrates. Eating an apple or a pear instead of a chocolate biscuit doesn't sound very enticing but it is a habit you ought to cultivate. In the end, the less refined sugar you consume the less you will want to eat it.

An alternative (although I think it is better to retrain your mind not to crave sugar first) is carob which, although rich in natural sugar, is also high in calcium and potassium, it contains no caffeine and hardly any fat and it has vitamins B1, B3 and A.

You can make a chocolate cake using less than two ounces of flour (see in recipe section) using bitter chocolate which has more than 60 per cent cocoa in it. I find it sweet enough - and that's saying something. You can also make a chocolate mousse which has no carbohydrates except those in the chocolate, so there is no need to deprive yourself forever and ever.

Fats

Sometimes called lipids, just to confuse you. But I'm sure you all know by now they are divided into two types: saturated fatty acids derived from animals (meat, fish, butter, cheese, cream etc.) And unsaturated or poly-unsaturated fatty acids which come from vegetable oils.

You do need some fat in your diet because it contains a number of essential vitamins, particularly A, D, E and K. But it is crucial to make sure fat constitutes less than 25 percent of your total daily intake of food.

Meat and dairy products are all perfectly healthy so long as you don't eat too much of them. The recommended daily intake for men is 90 grams and for women 70 grams of which no more than 10 per cent should be saturates although, if you eat 100 grams of ham, how much of that is fat and how much lots of other things, is rather complicated to work out. The message you need to take on board is eat fat frugally. It might help you if you tried to count up your fat intake for one day, just to see.

Since lipids are also responsible for cholesterol, they can be sub-divided again into "good" and "bad". Bad ones include those found in saturated fat but good ones can help to lower cholesterol and these include olive and corn oils, rape seed oil and sunflower margarines, salmon, sardines, pilchards, herrings, kippers and mackerel. There is general agreement among scientists now that if you eat at least two oily fish dishes a week you will be doing your heart a favour.

Fibre

The Committee on Medical Aspects of Food Policy (COMA) which works out these things, says we should be eating an average of 18 grams of fibre a day. It is found mainly in vegetables, fruit and whole cereals although for obvious reasons, if you are on a diet, it makes more sense to bulk out your meals with huge helpings of cabbage which has so many other good things in it, than a cereal which may have rather a lot of carbo-hydrates.

Although it has no energy value, insoluble fibre (which used to be called roughage) fulfils a number of functions. The cellulose, lignin, pectin and gums contained by fibre help to maintain a healthy digestive system and prevent constipation. It also helps to prevent gallstones. Although fibre passes through the system without being absorbed, it scoops up harmful waste products on its travels.

Fibre is rich in vitamins and trace elements and can limit the toxic effects of some chemical substances such as food additives and colourings. On the other hand bran, wholewheat pasta, and large amounts of wholemeal bread contain phytic acid, a substance which blocks the absorption of calcium, magnesium, iron, zinc, copper and vitamin B—another reason for choosing the fruit and vegetable option.

Soluble fibre is thought to have a role in helping to delay the absorption of sugar and also assists in keeping blood cholesterol levels down.

Sources are wholegrains and all the products made from them like bread, porridge oats and sweet corn; all fruit (raspberries have the most fibre), then pears, apples, strawberries, peaches (eaten with the skin on where feasible); vegetables such as green peas, parsley, artichoke, leeks, cabbage, mushrooms and potatoes, although the processing of potatoes into chips lowers their fibre content.

Fish

Most people who are interested in their health eat plenty of fish but how many eat enough oily fish? Herrings, pilchards, sprats, sardines, mackerel, trout, untinned tuna and salmon are some you should be eating at least two or three times a week.

Beside being a useful ingredient in the fight to ward off heart disease by helping to reduce LDL cholesterol level by aiding in the blood's fluidity, oily fish can improve serious skin disorders, including eczema and psoriasis.

They can also help arthritis sufferers: two of our six guinea pigs in Broadbottom suffer from serious arthritis. The fatty acids in fish oils can be converted by our cells into anti-inflammatory agents, easing joint pain and stiffness. Obviously, losing weight is also important because if joints are carrying excess fat, that is a strain on the mechanism.

White fish is low in fat but high in vitamins and minerals

Herbs

It is essential, especially when you are dieting, to sprinkle your food with herbs either during cooking or afterwards, because nothing defeats a dieter more than eating bland meals. If you train yourself to use herbs and spices frequently you will soon appreciate how much more interesting food can be. The problem with the kind of food that makes us fat is that it is so over-loaded with sugar or salt our taste buds become distorted and it isn't easy to wean them onto more subtle flavours.

The reason herbs are so aromatic is they store a high concentration of essential oils from one per cent in thyme to 15 per cent in cloves. These do you good in hundreds of different ways so you should use as wide a variety as possible. Garlic, fennel and mint are well-known aids to digestion. Sage derives its name from the Latin verb salvere—to heal—and was in common use for centuries before the Romans brought it to Britain. Chives are a common herb to add to salads and dill, especially added to tomatoes or a dressing, is equally delicious. Sweet marjoram adds flavour to meat and poultry—drizzle meat with olive oil, sprinkle the marjoram over and rub it in gently then let it marinade for a few hours. Grow herbs yourself if you can. But if you can't get them fresh, dried herbs will do.

Meat

Does anyone today still need telling that too much red meat is bad for you? I doubt it. Our friends in Broadbottom certainly received that message many years ago and hardly any of them has red meat more than twice a week now. There have been innumerable studies showing its ill effects on the heart and being implicated in fatal cancers. A recent one, conducted in America by the Harvard School of Public Health over a four-year period, followed the diets of over 47,855 men aged 40 to 75. It found that even if men don't change their eating habits until later in life, they can still significantly reduce the risk of suffering from prostate cancer.

Having said all that, most of us do like our red meat and I wouldn't dream of suggesting you never eat it again. A grilled sirloin steak with a green salad is one of my own favourite meals. But I am happy to eat it only occasionally rather than regularly because, besides being healthier, it makes it more of a treat.

As a general rule, your daily intake of food should be divided up like this: 5 portions from the fruit and vegetable group, 4 from the cereals and potato group, 2 portions from the meat and alternatives group (including fish and eggs) and 2 from the milk and milk products group (which should include at least half a pint of milk a day for drinks and cereals).

Proteins

Protein is needed to produce blood corpuscles, secrete hormones, produce scar tissue and maintain muscle tone. Proteins are the organic cells that make up living matter and are made up of simpler bodies called amino acids. Some amino acids are produced by the body but mostly we get what we want from food.

There is no need to worry about not getting enough protein - in the Western world many of our ills stem from a diet that is over-loaded with protein. All we need to consume is about three ounces a day. You get protein mainly from animal sources—meat, fish, cheese, eggs and milk—or vegetables like soybean and nuts.

A popular diet is to follow a high protein, low carbohydrate regime. It does mean you are never hungry because you can eat vast amounts of, for instance, cooked chicken, but I am wary of this type of diet. By eating only protein you can also be taking in too much fat and losing too much water. Carbohydrate turns into glycogen which binds water and as soon as you re-introduce starch into your diet, your body replenishes its glycogen store. But mucking about drastically with your system is never a good idea. Also, if your physical activity is low, unburned protein residues will stay in the body and be transformed into uric acid which can cause other problems, including gout. None of our Broadbottom dieters opted for a protein-only diet because what we were aiming for was a healthy eating plan they could adopt for life—not just a quick fix for now.

Pulses

Pulses are something you will learn to turn to, if you haven't already, as you reduce the amount of meat you eat and start learning about how to feed your body in the most healthy way possible. Although dried lentils, peas and beans still retain some of their old-fashioned image—that is, that they are bland, cheap and therefore second class and "difficult" to cook—more and more people are taking a deep breath and plunging into pulses. It is a rewarding experience. Both Carol and Andrew are fans and constantly surprise themselves with the versatility of their inventions. They also swear their families are healthier as a result of eating more pulse-based meals.

Although pulses are generally grown in warm, temperate climates, strenuous efforts are being made by research establishments in this country to find a way of growing them here. Since we are massive importers of lentils, peas and beans, it would make sense not only for our farming community but for the economy as a whole. Especially since there are hundreds of health writers like me, preaching the gospel according to pulses and converting many more thousands of people all the time. Environmentalists are keen on pulses, too, not least because they are "nitrogen fixing" which means they leave the soil richer than they found it.

They contain about 80 calories per ounce (28 g) and as well as providing a cheap source of protein, with the lowest amount of fat, they contain iron, phosphorus and B vitamins. Their fibre content is extremely high, which adds to their healthy credentials. Unfortunately, I think their "roughage" reputation has been over-stated to the extent that a lot of people think they are a useful addition to, say, soup but produce so much wind they are generally not worth the effort. This is a shame because if you prepare them properly, pulses don't have to produce any embarrassing side effects.

Basically, preparation consists of four processes: washing, soaking, rinsing and cooking, with an extra parboiling-and-rinsing before the final cooking if you find it's necessary to make them digestible.

Salt

A lot of fuss has been made about salt in the last ten years and not all the information is accurate. What is true is that there is plenty of salt in food already, so you don't need to add any. Vegetables ought always to be eaten raw or steamed, so the question of adding salt to the boiling water should not arise.

There may be a connection between salt and water retention and salt and blood pressure. So, to be on be safe side, cut down on salt. But beware of buying a substitute: it is not the answer, often causing as many problems as the original. If you have a craving for salt, it could be because you are deficient in zinc, according to some experts who recommend you cut out salt and take a 15mg zinc supplement instead. Otherwise, learn to flavour your food with spices as a tasty alternative.

Sugar

Start cutting out all the skull-and-crossbones symbols you come across and stick them onto your packets of sugar, jars of jam and tins of biscuits. Yes, sugar is that dangerous.

Confectionery, fizzy drinks and all the rest of the goodies we consume which contain refined sugar place undue stress on the pancreas. It is the job of the pancreas to keep the body's level of insulin stable—but how can it function satisfactorily if it is constantly being plied with sugar the body was not designed to accommodate?

Our bodies don't need refined sugar at all. We survived very well without it for thousands of years, until it began to be produced commercially in the eighteenth century. It contains no nutrients whatsoever and creates havoc resulting, for many people, in listlessness, mood swings, depression, hostility, fearfulness, crying spells, false feelings of food cravings, hypertension, dizzy spells and confusion—besides contributing, eventually, to obesity. As if that wasn't enough, sugar contributes to diabetes, gastritis, ulcers, bad teeth and heart problems.

There are three types of sugar that effect the amount of blood glucose in our body, expressed in terms of a glyceamic index. The highest level would occur after eating glucose itself followed very closely by honey which raises the level to within 10 per cent of pure glucose. Then there is fructose (fruit sugar) which contains no glucose and is converted slowly into glucose by the liver and causes only a small percentage rise in the glyceamic index. And lastly there is sucrose, which includes all refined sugar. It is 50 per cent glucose and 50 per cent fructose and you don't need to be a mathematician to work out that those foods would make the index rise 50 percent. A Mars Bar would be 60 on the index, dark chocolate (with more than 60 per cent cocoa) 22. Even carrots are way up there at 85, so if you are seriously trying to wean yourself away from food which sends your pancreas into a see-saw mode, you could do worse than learn the glycaemic index table off by heart.

Fresh fruit and berries contain natural sugar (fructose) plus a range of vitamins, minerals and fibre. So they are safe - just so long as you don't add sugar, of course!

Approximately 16 per cent of our calorie intake is from sugar and of that, 80 per cent comes hidden in processed food. The other 20 per cent we tip on our cornflakes or into our coffee and tea. Knowingly, willingly, foolishly.

Experts think we should cut down our intake by 50 per cent. I think we should cut it down by 90 per cent.

Cravings for sweet treats can be the body's way of signalling that its blood glucose level is low. The trouble is, feeding it with a sugary snack instead of something more sensible will make the level rise temporarily. But it will only be a quick fix and you will be "hungry" again shortly afterwards. It's boring but true that the highs and lows of refined sugar consumption do you a lot of harm both physically and mentally.

Dates are the sweetest of all dried fruits, containing over 50 percent natural fruit sugar as well as fibre, calcium, iron, potassium and phosphorous —and would therefore be a healthier alternative to chocolate. Figs and prunes have a gentle laxative property and are also high in natural fruit sugars. But they are high in calories, so should be kept out of the house until you have reached your target weight. By then you will have learned how to control those harmful cravings.

As a basic guide to healthy—and slimming— eating, follow these guidelines:
CUT OUT
All fried food
Lard, dripping
Red meat
Pork and lamb
Processed meats, sausages, corned beef,
Cream
Sauces: white, tomato, brown, mayonnaise
Butter
Full cream milk
Alcohol
Sugar, sweets, chocolate, fizzy drinks
Cereals with sugar coatings
Biscuits, cakes, pies, pastries
Tinned vegetables
Tinned fruit, jam, marmalades

Full fat cheese

CUT DOWN
Margarine
Oil
Pasta
Rice
Low-cal cheese
Poultry
White bread
Nuts
Processed food

EAT UP
Vegetables - raw or steamed
Fruit
Skimmed milk
Chicken without the skin
Fish, especially oily fish
Cottage cheese

DRINK UP
Water
Juice - tomato, orange, grapefruit etc

Alcohol

There is a difference between addiction and craving. A craving does not occur very often and once it has been satisfied you should not get the same feeling for a long time. An addiction, on the other hand, is insatiable. You become a slave to it. Which category best describes your liking for alcohol? For most of us, thank goodness, alcohol is just something we like to drink, usually at the end of the day. The trouble is, alcohol contains an awful lot of calories—so many, you may not have to diet at all, just go on the wagon for a while.

If you drink too much, the liver won't function efficiently and it is the liver which is the major filter for the bloodstream, preventing toxins from reaching other vital organs.

It also blocks absorption of essential nutrients, particularly vitamins B and C, magnesium and zinc. And because it is a diuretic, it causes further loss of vitamins.

Levels of oestrogen in women and testosterone in men are reduced by heavy drinking and it can lead to irregular periods or lowered libido. Some people are allergic to yeast so can be made quite ill by drinking beer. It can also make asthma worse—and it stimulates the appetite.

Too much alcohol has a harmful effect on the cardiovascular system and induces arterial hypertension. On the other hand, studies have shown that two units of alcohol a day can help to reduce the risk of heart disease and cholesterol gallstone formation. But that means 2 four-ounce glasses of wine or just under 1 pint of beer—nothing like getting legless on a regular basis.

Smoking

Beside being incredibly bad for your lungs and heart (tobacco is the cause of 25 per cent of cardiovascular disease), smoking cigarettes is unhealthy because they are full of chemicals which the body regards as poisonous foreign bodies, namely toxins. When they are not eliminated, these toxins may find themselves dumped in your fat stores, out of harm's way. From the body's point of view, fat is a safe place to put poisons because it is the least metabolically active tissue so can't do too much harm to other vital organs. The trouble is, when you start dieting, the fat is brought out of storage and the toxins come with it.

Smoking deadens the taste buds and some people insist it also deadens their appetite, although there are plenty of overweight smokers. Unfortunately many people, especially women, are convinced they will put on weight if they give up smoking which is ludicrous when you think about it. They will put on weight if they substitute sweets for cigarettes, obviously, but there's no law that says smokers have to replace one bad habit with another. I am convinced, if you listen to the hypnosis tape regularly, the message that you and your body will be in tune with each other, will eventually gnaw away at the nicotine fix because our bodies must hate it. It's the mind that is playing the temptress while the poor body has to suffer the consequences.

Water

Whether you are on a diet or not, you should drink two litres of water every day. Not the sparkling kind because it isn't a good idea to put more gas into your body. Nor is it good for your digestive system to drink while you eat— rather try to drink a large glass of water well before your meal. If your local water tastes good and you are confident about the quality, fill a bottle and keep it in the fridge—that way you will know how much you have to get through. Add lemon, lime or sprig of mint to give it extra taste. You might like to copy one tip I had from a doctor friend: she makes a one litre pot of "tea" twice a day and drinks it all up before bedtime. She pours boiling water onto half a lemon and grates half a tea-spoon of ginger root into it. It acts like a gentle scourer.

LITTLE THINGS MEAN A LOT

Vitamins are organic substances which play a vital role in our overall health. They are enablers, working to keep the body functioning properly. As everyone is different, each person's needs will depend on what his or her body requires at different times, how they metabolise their food, what extra calls are being made on their system by their diet or lifestyle. The only sensible way to make sure you do not suffer from a vitamin deficiency is to eat as varied a diet as possible, so you are feeding your body with all the extra ingredients it requires. If you do think you are lacking in a particular vitamin, be your own doctor-detective and find out which food contains it. Then you can include more in your diet or take a supplement. That doesn't mean to say more is better. A multi-vitamin which contains all the recommended daily amount of nutrients is probably your safest bet.

Although most of us in this country are lucky and we no longer suffer from serious vitamin deficiencies, a lack of certain vitamins can cause a whole host of minor ailments. This probably applies ten times more to smokers than non-smokers because the toxins in cigarettes will often counteract the benefits of vitamins and trace minerals. The same goes for heavy drinkers and even people who drink excessive amounts of tea and coffee may find they are deficient in essential vitamins because of the damaging effects of caffeine.

What is exciting today about vitamins is the scientific research coming to light which proves that some can have a significant impact on preventing serious diseases developing. These include cancers, heart attacks and cataracts.

The vitamins which can help are called antioxidants. Beta-carotene, the substance which gives some fruit and vegetables their bright yellow or orange colour, or produces the very dark green of some cabbages and lettuce, is one. Other antioxidants are vitamins C and E.

Imagine your body is a war zone and zooming around it like loose cannons are things called free radicals which attack healthy cells. Free radicals are molecules generated as part of the body's normal process. Usually they are arranged in pairs, this pairing giving them stability. The trouble is, they can be made unstable by our modern environment. Oxidation—the same process that makes cars go rusty or butter go rancid—turns these harmless atoms into lethal weapons.

Pollution, pesticides, cigarette smoke, alcohol, the metabolism of certain drugs, food additives and ultra-violet radiation from the sun as a result of the ozone layer getting thinner, can all boost the number of loose free radicals being produced in our bodies today. They cause a chain reaction, damaging the walls of our cells which causes substances to ooze out, creating all kinds of damage and mayhem depending on what is leaking where.

The body has its own inbuilt defence system of antioxidants which prevents further oxidation and therefore guards cells against free radical damage. But it makes sense, since we breathe in so much potential damage these days, to give ourselves extra protection by eating the right food and including extra doses of antioxidants in our daily diet.

According to the latest government survey of diet and nutrition among British adults, the daily intake of beta-carotene is about two milligrams whereas many expert organisations such as the United States National Cancer Institute (NCI) are recommending a diet that would provide six milligrams of beta-carotene per day.

To get the most out of beta-carotene, because it is a fat-soluble nutrient, you need, for instance, a knob of butter with your boiled carrots. (And, incidentally, boiled carrots provide more beta-carotene than raw ones.) The mayonnaise in coleslaw does the same job. But don't think that gives you licence to use lashings of fat. It doesn't—too much fat causes other serious problems.

There is no mystery about why vitamins are called A, B, C and so on. It is simply the order in which they were first discovered.

Vitamin A is one of the most important, essential for growth, healthy skin and good eyesight, especially night vision. It also helps to reinforce the protective membrane surrounding cells, which is why it is so crucial in fighting free radicals. In particular, it helps to protect against infection of the nose, throat, lungs and urinary tract.

There are two main types of vitamin A: retinol, found in animal foods like meat and dairy products and carotenoids, found in fruit and vegetables. There are hundreds of those but the most important is beta-carotene. Liver and fish liver oils are rich sources of vitamin A, so are carrots, eggs, cheese, milk, sweet potatoes, spring greens and spinach.

Vitamin B is one of the most complex vitamins and plays a vital role in releasing energy from the cells. Stress quickly depletes the body's store of vitamin B which translates into anxiety, irritability and depression.

Vitamin B is broken down into a series of numbers—B1, B2, B3, B5, B6 and B12—and you may, at any one time, find you lack one or even more of the B complex group. Pregnant women who have already had a pregnancy affected by a neural tube defect and may be at risk of giving birth to a spina bifida baby, are recommended to take supplements of folic acid, one of the B complex vitamins, before they become pregnant.

Folic acid is particularly vulnerable to heat and air so a supplement is often advisable. It is found in large quantities in brewer's yeast so a yeast extract either as a hot drink or on toast is a good item to include in your daily diet. Folic acid is also to be found in wheatgerm, nuts, pig's liver, pulses, green leafy vegetables, wholemeal bread and eggs.

The main cause of vitamin B1—thiamin—deficiency is alcoholism. It is needed for the release of energy from carbohydrates, fats and alcohol and the more of those you eat or drink, the more thiamin you need. It is water-soluble and is one of the vitamins most affected by cooking.

Emotionally unstable individuals are often found to suffer from a thiamin deficiency and a whole range of illnesses are claimed to be alleviated by taking a supplement, including lumbago, sciatica and facial paralysis. Good sources include yeast extract, brown rice, nuts, pork, cod's roe, lentils, wholemeal bread and pasta and fortified breakfast cereals.

Vitamin B2—riboflavin—releases energy from other foods and is found mainly in meat and milk. But because it is destroyed by exposure to light, milk left on the doorstep, even in cold weather, will lose all its B2 content. If you suffer from mouth ulcers, a lack of riboflavin in your diet could be the reason. Eyes can also be affected with burning, itchiness and visual fatigue occurring where there is not sufficient B2. Again, yeast extract is a good source, so is lamb's liver, pig's kidney and fortified breakfast cereal.

Vitamin B3—niacin—like the other B vitamins is water soluble, though it is more stable than the others, being unaffected by light, air or alkalis.

It is involved in blood circulation, maintenance of the nervous system and the reduction of cholesterol and fats as well as energy production.

Symptoms of niacin deficiency are tiredness, depression and loss of memory. Sources are real coffee, poultry, liver, oily fish like sardines, herrings, mackerel and kippers, bacon, eggs, pork, cheddar cheese, frozen peas and wholemeal bread.

Vitamin B5—pantothenic acid—plays an important part in the process of releasing energy from fat, carbohydrates and protein and is widely available in both animal and vegetable foods. It is destroyed by heat, vinegar or bicarbonate of soda and leaks into cooking water.

B5 is crucial to the functioning of the adrenal gland and in the formation of antibodies and as a nutritional supplement can help the body to cope with stress. It may also help to reduce allergic reactions in the respiratory and digestive systems.

Dieters who want to blame their metabolism for their weight problem should bear in mind that vitamin B6—pyridoxine—assists with the metabolism of proteins. Some claims have also been made that it helps to alleviate premenstrual tension but there is no conclusive evidence for this. However, if you suffer badly it may be worth trying a supplement for a while to see if it makes a difference. Too high doses can be dangerous, so don't overdo it.

Vitamin B6 converts protein into energy and plays a role in the production of red blood cells and hormone production. It is found in bacon, liver, oats, pulses, oranges, bananas and poultry.

Vitamin B12—cobalamin—contains cobalt, hence its name. It is essential for the formation of red blood cells and unlike most of the other vitamins, the body can store excess quantities of B12 in the liver. Unfortunately, the downside of that is it might take years for a vitamin B12 deficiency to show up when pernicious anaemia could result in irreversible neurological damage.

Vegans are particularly at risk as vitamin B12 does not normally occur in vegetables. Alcoholics are also susceptible. Good sources include lamb and pig's liver, white fish, cod's roe, yoghurt and oysters.

Vitamin C—ascorbic acid—is probably the best known vitamin and has a lot of important functions. It is especially helpful in warding off coughs and colds during the winter but, less commonly known, it helps to make collagen, the substance that binds the cells of our tissues. It also helps wounds to heal quickly. It is associated with relieving stress, offering protection from infection and acting as a natural anti-histamine.

The body cannot manufacture its own vitamin C, nor does it store it up for future use, so it should be taken daily by eating the right food, like lots of oranges. Or, if you think a vitamin C booster is called for, in the form of a supplement.

Its basic function is to help with the growth and repair of bones, teeth, gums and body tissues. But it is also involved in the body's immune system which is why it is reckoned to be such a useful ally in fighting off flu symptoms. It also plays a crucial part in the formation of antibodies and the stimulation of white blood cells and also helps with the metabolism of folic acid.

The latest expert opinion is that we should be eating between 60-100 milligrams of vitamin C a day. Since heat destroys this vitamin, as many fruits and vegetables as possible should be eaten raw. (But anyway, always steam vegetables and if you do boil them in water, save the water, if you can, to add to soup or for making gravy or a sauce.) A jacket potato will contain twice as much vitamin C as peeled and boiled potatoes.

Light and air also destroy vitamin C so vegetables and fruit should be stored in a cool, dark cupboard and eaten as soon as possible. Good sources include blackcurrants, kiwi fruit, sprouts, mango, cauliflower, cabbage, strawberries, citrus fruits, peas (but not dried boiled ones) tomato (raw or juice), bananas and milk.

Vitamin D—calciferol—is converted in the body to a hormone needed for the absorption of calcium. It is essential for the healthy growth of bones and teeth and is often referred to as the sunshine vitamin because we get it from daylight (though not sunbathing). Sources rich in vitamin D are cod liver oil, herrings, mackerel, sardines and kippers, dairy products and margarine which is fortified with vitamin D by law.

Vitamin E—tocopherol—is a powerful nutrient which protects the lipids in cell walls. Lipids are particularly susceptible to oxidation by free radicals. Oxidative damage resulting from free radical attack has been linked to the onset of premature ageing, cancer, atherosclerosis, cataracts and an array of degenerative diseases.

Since vitamin E's discovery in 1922, it has been nicknamed the 'virility vitamin' because it is closely associated with fertility. It is essential for maintaining a healthy immune system: it helps to protect the eyes, skin, liver, breast and calf muscle tissues as well as helping to prevent tumour growth.

It also protects the lungs from oxidative damage and can act to reduce the oxygen requirement of muscles and so increase exercise capacity. You obtain vitamin E from oils such as wheatgerm, safflower, sunflower, cod liver and olive, almonds, asparagus, spinach, broccoli, butter, peanut butter, bananas, tomato puree, raw egg yolk and strawberries.

Vitamin K is sometimes called nature's Elastoplast because it helps to prevent bleeding. Vitamin K deficiency is rare because it is widespread in the food chain, in vegetables and dairy produce, and because bacteria in the gut synthesises much of what we need. But lack of it may become a problem for people on extended courses of antibiotics or very low calorie diets. Bruising easily can be a sign of vitamin K deficiency.

MINERALS

Calcium is the most abundant mineral in the human body, found mostly in bones and teeth. Vegetarians and especially vegans may be at risk of calcium deficiency and young women with a history of osteoporosis in the family need to make sure their diet includes plenty of calcium-carrying foods like milk, cheese, yoghurt and white bread—which often has calcium added, making it more healthy from that point of view than wholemeal bread. Sardines, white fish, roasted peanuts and eggs also contain calcium.

Magnesium, along with calcium and phosphorus, provides the bones with structure and strength. It is also involved in the process of breaking down food for energy and in the smooth working of nerves and muscles. Magnesium supplements are often taken by women who suffer from PMT, especially if they have stomach cramps and sugar cravings. Food sources include peanuts, plain chocolate, cheese, chicken, white fish, oranges and potatoes.

Iron gives red blood cells their colour and transports oxygen round the body. It is essential to prevent anaemia which causes tiredness, lack of stamina, pallor and breathlessness. Although it is important, iron is only a trace mineral in terms of concentration in the body. It is estimated that ten per cent of women between 18-50 have low stores of iron so it is particularly important if you think you are likely to be one of the ten per cent, that you make sure you eat some iron-rich foods at least twice a week. These include fortified breakfast cereals, lamb's liver and pig's kidneys, dried apricots, nuts, seafood, corned beef and plain chocolate. For obvious reasons, if you're providing yourself with some of the above for their iron content, you have to be particularly careful you don't over-dose on the calorie front!

Potassium plays a part in controlling the fluid level in the body and long-term use of certain antibiotics, especially penicillin, may deplete the sup-ply. It is kept inside the cell and is counter-balanced by sodium which remains outside the cell and can aggravate fluid retention. Most of our sodium comes as salt added to food in preparation and there is a lot of conflicting information about how much salt we eat and its effect on slim-ming. According to one expert we consume .35-.45 ounces of salt daily when our bodies only need .10-.14 ounces. All I suggest is you cut down as much as possible. Don't add salt to the food on your plate or when you are cooking because we generally get plenty without even trying. One gram of salt makes you retain 100 grams of water: if you look carefully at the ingredients of a whole range of food—tinned meat, bacon, sausages, crisps, wholemeal bread, cheddar cheese, yeast and beef extracts—you'll see they all have an abundance of salt in them already. Buy potassium salt and steer clear of gravy brownings if you think water retention is a particular problem.

Zinc is needed for growth and repair and is the mineral found most highly concentrated in the muscles, liver, kidneys and eyes. It also makes an important contribution to keeping our skin smooth, supple and blemish-free. During puberty there is an increased requirement for zinc due to increased hormone production and a zinc supplement can be an effective treatment for acne sufferers. It may also help people suffering from rheu-matoid arthritis because there is a link between zinc and essential fatty acid metabolism. Women on the contraceptive pill often have lower zinc levels than other women and sometimes pregnant women need a zinc supplement. Zinc plays a part in the production of over eighty enzymes and hormones in the body so a deficiency would have widespread effects. It is measured in milligrams (mg) and it is estimated that on average our daily intake is around 10.5 mg although some research claims the recom-mended daily allowance ought to be 15 mg. Many factors decrease the amount of zinc available for the body to use and people who smoke or drink heavily should consider taking a supplement. Zinc is found in calves' liver, red meat, poultry, sardines, cheese, brown rice and beans.

Selenium (the name comes from the moon goddess Selene) is a trace mineral but nevertheless is important in the prevention of liver disease and is an essential part of our diet. It helps to preserve normal liver function, offers protection against cancer and boosts the immune system by protecting our white blood cells. It also helps to prevent the harmful effects of potentially poisonous metals like arsenic, cadmium, mercury and lead. Good food sources are offal, shellfish, wholegrains and cereals, raw mushrooms and boiled eggs.

Chromium has only recently come to the fore in the slimming world with claims that chromium picolinate can increase the metabolic rate, suppress the appetite and cravings for sugar. If it does all that it would be a miracle! There are indications that it may be able to increase lean muscle mass in athletes and it helps to lower total cholesterol levels and increase beneficial high density lipoproteins (HDL) cholesterol. It is available in egg yolk, molasses, brewer's yeast, red meat and grape juice although you can also take is as a supplement, so long as you don't go over 25 micrograms daily.

GET UP AND GO!

Regular exercise is as important for your health as eating the right food. It is helpful in reducing cholesterol. It makes your heart and lungs stronger and makes your heart work more efficiently. It helps strengthen your muscles, joints and even your bones. It helps to lower blood pressure, to maintain and increase bone density. It improves your circulation and, contrary to what you might think, exercise actually makes you feel less tired. By taking regular exercise, especially after a stressful day, you'll find you sleep better—and it helps to lift depression or feelings of aggression. All that and it makes you look good, too.

Inactivity, on the other hand, leads to dodgy heart conditions or weak and brittle bones. What is also dangerous is that people who do not do any strenuous exercise are generally unaware how low their capacity is for sustained physical activity. Eventually they will discover that even climbing the stairs is an effort. And as for running for a bus or running in an emergency, forget it. Too often people don't bother until something terrible happens. They realise how overweight they are, they start getting the first twinges of arthritis or become seriously out of breath even when performing minor chores.

However, the good news is the bad news is reversible. Once they get up and go with regular exercise, people of any age can cope with longer and harder activity than they could before. And in a surprisingly short time. You will be amazed at how quickly your body responds to being pushed—gently at first, of course. But gradually you can increase exercise until your stamina becomes quite impressive.

For someone who wants to lose weight, doing regular exercise does you even more good. Because it raises your metabolic rate, exercise means you burn off more fat. So instead of storing food as fat, it gets used up as fuel to keep the body going. The rate you burn fat slows down as you get older and, of course, some people store fat more than others. So both groups have an added incentive for doing exercises. If the activity you take up is prolonged and undertaken regularly, your metabolic rate will rise even when you are resting.

Weight loss often levels out after you have been dieting for a while and that can be very depressing. A partial explanation seems to be that your metabolic rate falls during a period of calorie restriction. This is possibly a defensive mechanism brought into play instinctively by the body to preserve itself during periods of starvation. It may also be because you don't feel like being so physically active if you are eating less. But it is worth remembering that a programme of regular aerobic activity will increase energy consumption not only during the period of exercise but for several hours afterwards. One study shows that after 60 to 90 minutes of vigorous exercise, oxygen consumption was increased for at least the next 24 hours.

Doing a regular programme of exercises will help you to cope with everyday activities by strengthening your muscles. Following eight or ten weeks of an exercise training programme, physical effort can be sustained for longer and causes less fatigue. This effect is a result of physiological changes in the muscles and in the cardiovascular system.

Several biochemical changes occur to the muscles, besides an increase in strength and size. The number and density of the capillaries increases as does the activity of cellular enzymes, so improving oxygen supply and extraction. More fat is used in the process of oxidation and carbohydrates are broken down more effectively. In what is the opposite of a vicious circle—a positive circle, if you like—these metabolic changes probably reduce fatigue and discomfort in the exercising muscles because less lactic acid is produced. The thing to remember is it is dynamic rhythmic exercises like walking, running, cycling or swimming which bring about the necessary changes.

The exercise you choose does not have to be too vigorous but you do have to increase your heart rate over a period of 30 minutes at least three times a week. That means getting out of breath, but you can always take a short rest during the thirty minutes—you don't have to keep at it non-stop. At first, until you are fitter, stopping and starting again will be a great help.

A good way to start is to run for sixty seconds then walk for sixty seconds for five minutes. Then, when that's comfortable, do it for ten minutes, then fifteen minutes and so on. As you build up your stamina you will be able to run for longer and longer. But never overdo it—it's better to keep going, running/walking for longer, than tiring yourself out by running very fast for a shorter time. You'll be amazed at yourself, and very pleased, when, after six months, you look back at how unfit you once were.

That's another thing: don't set yourself unrealistic goals. Don't go signing up for a marathon before you've even started. A steady improvement is all you need to aim for.

One of the most important things about exercise is to do something you enjoy. If putting a video on and doing aerobics and hip humps in your front room suits you, fine. If you need company, join a class. If you need discipline, join a team. If you can ride a bicycle, which is brilliant exercise for nearly all your muscles, plot a number of journeys every week, ones you can cope with, which have a purpose, but which are quite taxing. If it's too wet to cycle, substitute a swim.

A brisk walk, with emphasis on the brisk, starting at 20 minutes every day and building up to as long as time will allow, will also raise your heart rate to the level needed before the fat starts getting burned off. Time is the one word you will probably find crops up again and again to stop you doing anything. Just remember this: your body needs it as much as the carpet needs vacuuming or the dishes need to be washed. And it is a job you can't delegate.

Whatever you choose the most important thing about exercise is to DO it.

Before you undertake an exercise programme, make sure you are aware of these important guidelines.
•It's vital you warm up your muscles first by doing some gentle stretching exercises so you don't get cramp or risk an injury. For the same reason, you should do do stretching ones at the end, too. There will be less strain on your ligaments and you won't put yourself out of action.
•After a few weeks you will find all your warm-up and cool-down exercises are much easier to do. And after eight to ten weeks you should begin to see, and feel, a change in your body shape.
•It's not true there is "no gain without pain" as Jane Fonda insisted. As far as exercising is concerned, the message is: "If it hurts, don't do it."
•We are often shorter at the end of the day than we were in the morning. This is because the muscles and structures that support the spine tire and

sag and we tend, unconsciously, to let ourselves droop as the day goes on. Also, our discs become thinner during the day. As we get older we reduce in height which is also due to shrinking of the discs between the vertebrae and to loss of tone and elasticity in the muscles.

•Before you invest in an exercise video, try and do it or at least watch it. Some will get on your nerves (the music, for instance, is often irritating) and others will simply not suit you.

•Jog on the spot for a count of 100 as often as you can. Buy a skipping rope. You'll find it tough at first but it's great exercise, which is why boxers do it so much. Stand on tiptoe and hold that position. Do it as least six times and feel your calf muscles working.

•Stamina is only one aspect of fitness. To get really fit you need to develop your strength and suppleness as well.

Now check out these questions and put a ring around either the Yes or No. A Yes means you would benefit from being more active.

Do you quickly get out of breath walking uphill or even on the flat?
Yes No

Do your legs ache or feel weak after you've climbed a couple of flights of stairs?
Yes No

Do you find it difficult to bend down and tie your shoelaces, or put your sock or tights on?
Yes No

Do you find it difficult to comb the back of your hair or pull a jumper off?
Yes No

Is it difficult for you to get out of an armchair or the bath?
Yes No

Once you have been exercising regularly for at least two months, check your progress by trying this test.

Choose a reasonably flat route of about one mile. You can measure the distance in your car or by using a map. It's worth getting this part right so ask for professional help (a local police station, or driving school, for instance) because it's easy to under-estimate a mile if you're not used to measuring distance.

Walking, running or using a combination of both, cover the mile as quickly as you can without getting uncomfortably breathless. It is likely to take between 10 and 20 minutes, so aim for a pace you can keep up. If you have any pain or discomfort, stop. If you are over 55 or have not exercised regularly until recently, and it's the first time you've taken the test, it is best to walk all the way.

Check your result with the figures in the box and repeat the test every month to monitor how you are getting on.

If swimming or cycling is your main activity and you are doing it regularly you will certainly be getting fitter but you may not notice much improvement in your walking or running, so don't be discouraged. This is simply because each activity uses different sets of muscles. You can devise a similar sort of test for cycling and swimming.

FITNESS TEST—How to check your progress

Minutes taken to cover the mile	*Stamina/ fitness*
20 or over	very unfit
15-20	unfit
12-15	fair
10-12	fit
10 or under	very fit

Here are a few basic and easy exercises you can do at home any time of the day when you have a few moments to spare.

INNER THIGH MUSCLES

1. Sit comfortably on the floor with your knees bent and the soles of your feet together, as close to your body as you can get them. Slowly, let your knees drop towards the floor until you feel the stretch in the inner thigh muscles. Hold for a count of 10.

2. Sit with your legs as wide apart as possible and your hands on the floor in front of you. Keeping your knees pointing towards the ceiling, lean forward from the hips until you feel a stretch along the inside and back of your thighs. Hold for a count of 16.

OUTER THIGH MUSCLES

1. Lie on your side, lower leg bent, resting on your lower arm with your other arm placed in front of you for support. Lift your upper leg as high as it will go, hold for a few seconds and lower. Do as many times as you can. Change to other side.

2. Stand holding onto something for support, your other hand on your waist, and raise your outer leg in front of you with knee bent and toe facing forward as high as you can. Do at least three times with both legs. Keep your back straight and the standing leg relaxed.

3. Hold a chair or table for support, hand on waist and lift your leg straight to the side as high as it will go and hold. Feel the stretch and repeat three times at first.

TUMMY TUNERS

1. Wherever you are, whenever you remember, pull in your stomach muscles. Think tall.

2. Lie on your back, both knees bent, your feet flat on the floor and hip-width apart.
  Rest your head in your left hand and your right hand on the right thigh.
  Pulling in your tummy muscles, slowly curl your head and shoulders off the floor to reach your right hand.
  Do this eight times, or as many as you can manage, swopping over to your right hand behind your head and reaching to your left hand on left thigh.

3. Lie on your back, knees bent and feet flat. Place your fingertips behind your head for support.

Keeping your elbows back and your tummy muscles in, curl up off the floor bringing your right knee up to meet your chin half way.

Do eight times, or as many as you can, with each leg.

Don't pull your head up, make your tummy muscles do the work.

4. Lie in the same position but with both hands behind your head and keeping both feet on the floor throughout.

Curl up off the floor as far as you can eight times. Keep your tummy as flat as you can.

BUM TRIMMERS

1. Wherever you are, whenever you remember, pull in your buttocks. Think of dying to spend a penny and having to hold it in! Don't forget to breathe. Hold for a count of 10 followed by four quick pull ins.

2. Lie on your back with your knees bent and feet firmly on the floor. Keep your tummy flat and your shoulders on the floor.

Raise your hips off the floor to make a straight line from your knees to your chest.

Remaining in that position, tighten then relax your buttocks. Do as many times as you like.

3. Lie on your back with your legs raised over your hips. Cross your feet and bend your knees over your chest.

Pull in your tummy muscles and curl your buttocks and lower back off the floor. Squeeze your knees in towards your chest.

Rest your hands on your ribs or on the floor to give you some push.

4. Lie flat on the floor with your hands under your forehead. Raise first one straight leg, then the other, as many times as you can.

5. Kneel on the floor, resting on your hands and elbows which should be shoulder width apart. Raise first one bent leg then the other, pushing your foot towards the back of your head.

LUSCIOUS LEGS

1. Put a hand on the wall or a chair for support. Clasp your foot and pull it back towards your buttocks as far as it will go. Feel the stretch down the front of your thigh. Hold for a count of eight for each leg.

2. Stand with your feet just over shoulder width apart, toes pointing in the same direction as your knees. Keeping your heels firmly on the ground, your back straight, slowly bend then straighten your legs. Do at least four times and bend lower once it becomes easy.

3. Hold the back of a chair for support. Keeping the supporting leg slightly bent, lift one knee up towards your chest, toe pointing downwards, then lower to a resting position. Turn and face in the opposite direction and repeat with the other leg. Keep your back straight and repeat at least four times each side.

4. Lie on your side with your head resting in your hand, bending your knee for balance, keeping the thigh in a straight line with your body.
   Bend your upper leg backwards and clasp your ankle with your free hand.
Gently ease the heel towards your buttock and hold for a count of 16.

5. Sit on a firm kitchen chair. Stand up, without using your hands and without leaning forward too much. Make sure your legs straighten completely. Sit down again and repeat. Gradually progress to just touching the chair instead of sitting down each time.

6. Stand at the bottom of a flight of stairs. Step up onto the first step, making sure you straighten both legs. Step down again. Do this with alternate legs for as long as you can stand it!

7. Stand with your feet together and your knees slightly bent. Spring up, landing with your feet comfortably apart and your knees still bent. Spring up again, landing with your feet together this time. Repeat as a continuous movement—apart-together, apart-together. Once you can do about 20 repeats you can knock off and have a drink—of water!

79

WAIST WHITTLERS

1. Stand with your feet shoulder-width apart, knees slightly bent. Bend one arm down the side of your body to your knee and slide the other hand up the other side to your armpit. Start with three either side then go up to as many as you like. Make sure you keep your body straight.

2. Stand with your feet shoulder-width apart, knees slightly bent and, keeping one hand on your waist, reach up and across your body with the other arm, hand trying to touch the ceiling. Repeat at least three times.

3. When you can do those two easily, stand with your feet much wider apart with your left hand on your hip. Bend your right leg until you feel a stretch in the inner thigh. Keeping your hips still and holding the inner thigh stretch, take your right arm up above your head and bend sideways to the left until you feel an additional stretch down your right side. Hold for a count of eight. Change over sides.

4. Place hands on waist and, keeping your shoulders and knees still, rotate your hips first one way then the other. Do at least twice each way.

UNKNOT YOUR SHOULDERS

1. Stand with your feet slightly apart and place your hands on the front of your thighs. Curve your shoulders round while breathing out. Then stand up straight, overlap your hands behind your back but without clasping them, and pull your arms back as far as you can, squeezing your shoulder blades together and opening up your chest. Hold for a few seconds and do it four times.

2. Stand with your feet shoulder-width apart and your toes pointing forwards. Keeping your hips facing forwards all the time, draw a circle with first one arm then the other. Brush your ear as your hand, palm outwards, goes round and down.

3. Make a circular movement with both arms, bending your knees as you

swing your arms down and stretching up on tiptoe to make the circle as large as possible.

4. Stand with your feet a comfortable distance apart and bend your arms touching your fists in front of you. Keeping your elbows bent, swing them back as far as you can, then bring them round to the front again. Imagine your bent arms are having to press against some force. Repeat 6 times.

5. Do a scissors movement with your arms outstretched in front of you, taking them back as far as you can. Do at least 12 times swopping which arm is on top as you bring them across your body.

6. Place your right hand on your right shoulder. Move your elbow forwards, up and back, in a circle. Repeat with your left elbow and continue on alternate sides.

7. Stand tall and relaxed. Stretching through your whole body, reach up towards the ceiling with your fingertips. Then, letting yourself bend at the hips and knees, slowly bring your hands down towards the floor, as far as is comfortable. Straighten up and repeat.

HIP HUMPS

1. Sit on the floor with your arms out in front of you and "walk" backwards for ten "steps" and forwards again. This will hurt like mad so you have to start with just a few and do more and more as you become more supple. It's brilliant for breaking down all that fat on your behind.

HIP 'N THIGH

1. Hold onto a chair and, with one knee slightly bent, other hand on hip, raise your leg to the side, hold for a moment and close. Do this at least six times with each leg and feel the muscle on the outside of your thighs and hips working. Squeeze the buttock muscles tightly and make sure the working knee faces forward.

2. Lie on your back propped up on your elbows, one knee bent and one

leg straight. Keep the lower back pushing into the floor and raise the straight leg to the height of the bent knee so they are parallel. Hold then lower. Repeat eight times with each leg.

3. Lie on your back and keep one leg bent with foot flat on the floor. Bend the other leg into your body and clasp it with both hands, pulling it towards your body. Hold for a count of 16 for each leg.

4. Lie on your stomach on the floor. Slowly lift your right leg away from the floor as far as it will comfortably go. Slowly relax down and repeat with the other leg.

GENERAL STRENGTH BUILDERS

1. Stand at arm's length from a wall. Place your hands shoulder-width apart on the wall. Now bend your arms until your forehead touches the wall. Then push yourself away again until your arms are straight.

2. Kneel on all fours. Move your hands forward slightly and take most of your weight onto them. Bend your arms and lower the top half of your body towards the floor. Only go as far as is comfortable and be careful not to sag in the middle. Straighten your arms again and return to the starting position.

3. If you can do the kneeling press ups easily you may be ready to attempt a full press-up. Follow the instructions above but alter the starting position by lifting your knees off the floor, so that your weight is supported on your hands and toes and your body is in a straight line.

4. Lie on your back with your knees bent. Put your hands on the top of your thighs. Lifting just your head and shoulders off the floor, slide your fingers along your thighs as far as is comfortable. Then uncurl slowly back to the lying position. As an alternative you can do this exercise lying on your back with your feet and lower legs on the seat of a chair.

5. Lie on your stomach on the floor, with your arms at your sides, your shoulders relaxed and your head on one side. Slowly lift your head, neck

and shoulders away from the floor, turning your head so you are looking at the floor with your chin tucked in. Only go as far as is comfortable. Slowly relax down turning your head to the other side and repeat.

BE IN THE SWIM

I am not trying to persuade you to get physically fit just so your body looks better, although that is a welcome side effect. There are twin pressures on us today which make fitness a crucial factor in our well being. Generally most of us lead less active lives than our ancestors did and we suffer from more stress.

What you should be aiming for is more suppleness, strength and stamina and swimming is one of the best ways to achieve all three. The buoyancy of water helps immeasurably to achieve a wider range of movements. And because it offers resistance, you can strengthen your muscles with far less effort than it takes on dry land.

It is especially beneficial for people who are overweight because the body in water becomes virtually weightless. So you don't have that terrible strain fat people normally associate with exercise.

There are other benefits, too. For instance, there is less chance of straining your muscles and damaging ligaments or joints. Water cushions the body so when you do exercises lying on your back the spine is cradled in the water, unlike when you're lying on the floor, where support is rigid.

There is probably a swimming pool near you where they have regular aquarobics classes you can join. But you can also learn a few simple exercises to do on your own. Even if you can't swim, the beauty of doing exercises in water is that you don't need to be able to swim.

Many exercises can be carried out at the shallow end and once you gain confidence in the water, you can go deeper, until your shoulder are submerged. There is nothing wrong, though, with staying at the shallow end within clutching distance of the bar at the side. Many people who suffer from asthma, or who have a fear of water, feel much safer doing that. The important thing is to make a regular commitment to go to a swimming pool, then you will soon discover how much benefit you can get.

The most simple exercise is to run, which will warm you up as well as do the business. You can go from one side of the pool to the other or simply run on the spot holding onto the side if need be. If you can't join a class, try going with a friend because you can feel a bit of a lemon jumping up and down on the spot on your own! Having said that, I always go on my own and just get on with it. Who cares?

There are lots of exercises you can do. The trick is to choose which ones you like and to concentrate on those areas of your body which you feel need most attention. For most of us that means working on the waist, hips and legs. But because I spend so much of my time writing, I need to loosen up my shoulders regularly so I always include plenty of exercises to do that. Doing the back crawl is one of the best ways, I find, and if you can't swim, once you have confidence in the water, you can put your toes underneath the bar, lie on the water and just do the arm movements without going anywhere.

If you have arthritis anywhere you should see if there is professional help available (some pools have physiotherapists giving lessons) but I'm sure you will find underwater exercises will help.

You can wiggle your fingers, make circles with your wrists and shoulders, move knee joints—all much, much easier in water.

The first time I did underwater exercises was at a health farm about twenty years ago. I did them conscientiously for a few weeks then gradually kept forgetting what I was supposed to do. So eventually I sat down and wrote a brief description of them and put it inside a waterproof cover. I used to place this by the side of the pool to remind me what I should do next. A few people used to give me funny looks occasionally but my memory is so lousy I didn't see any way round it. Maybe it's an idea you'll want to copy.

Although I have suggested how many repeats you should do for some of the exercises, obviously this is entirely up to you. Never do more than you think you can handle and work out a routine for yourself that feels right.

Start gently, you have all the time in the world. By this time next year you could be as supple as a fish!

WARM UPS AND COOL DOWNS

These exercises are good for getting you going and also a good way to round off your routine.

Walk sideways, pushing the water away with your hands. Start with your hands together straight in front, then take them to the sides, like a breast stroke. Take four steps to begin with, although you will quickly be able to do more. Do the same number to the left.

Run forwards then backwards at least eight steps at a time.

Jog on the spot bringing your knees up as high as you can.

Stand, with knees slightly bent, feet planted firmly on the bottom of the pool. Keep one knee bent and straighten first one leg then the other out and to the side, toes of the leg you are straightening turned upwards, stretching your muscles in the forward leg. Do alternate legs at a fairly brisk pace. At the same time, clench your fists and bring them up towards your body, up and down in time to the leg movements.

MAKE A SPLASH

Hold the bar with one hand and steady yourself with the other hand on the side of the pool and bicycle for as long as you can.

Holding onto the bar with your elbows against the side for balance and standing close to the wall, do a scissors movement with your legs pushing them as wide as possible.

Lie on the water and try to touch the bottom of the pool with alternate feet.

Holding onto the bar and lying on top of the water, kick with both feet behind you. Make as much of a splash as you can, moving your whole leg, not just your feet. You may need to place one hand on the side of the pool for balance. Do as many as you can. Work up to 20 each time. It's great for legs, stomach and waist.

Do the same but lying on the water facing upwards. Give the movement some force.

ON THE SPOT

Holding the side, lie on the water and make circular movements with your ankles both clockwise and anti-clockwise. Repeat at least 6 times each.

Standing with your back to the water lift one leg sideways as far as you can at least 4 times to begin with. Repeat with the other leg.

Stand with your heels against the side of the pool, feet flat on the bottom and, facing the water, put your hands back to clutch the bar. Then let yourself lean into the pool. Move your hands as close together as you can.

Hold onto the side with your left hand and stand firmly on your left leg. Lift the right leg in front to about knee height, keeping your foot bent. Circle the leg to the side and back and then push through close to the left leg. This should be a strong, fairly fast and low circling movement taken with strong pressure against the water throughout.

In the same position, swing the leg as far forwards and upwards towards the surface of the water as you can and then swing it backwards, taking the leg close to the supporting foot. Perform eight complete swings and repeat with the other leg, making your swings as high as possible.

STRETCHING

Hold the bar with both hands and walk up the side of the pool until your feet and hands are as close together as you can get them. Hold the position. You will feel your spine and the backs of your legs stretching. Do this every so often.

Hold the bar with your left hand and keep your left foot on the floor of the pool with your leg straight but not stiff. Bring your right leg back so your heel is touching your bottom and hold the ankle with your right hand. Feel the stretch down the front of your thigh. Keep legs close together and hold for a count of eight. Repeat three or four times each leg.

At the shallow end, hold the bar and keep both feet firmly on the floor. Bend one knee slightly and take the other leg back, still keeping the heel flat. You will feel the pull down the back of the straight leg. Hold for a count of eight and repeat as often as you can.

TWISTING

Holding onto the side and facing the pool, bring your knees up so you are in a sitting position and swing them from side to side. Twist so your knees go as close to the wall on either side as you can get them but try not to move your shoulders. Push hard against the water and grip a float between your knees to increase the resistance. Do eight times.

Facing the wall, bring your knees up to your chest then, keeping your ankles together, let them drop and push up your straight legs up behind you. Repeat, curling your knees up again and repeat four times. Pull in your stomach muscles as you bring your knees up.

Standing with your shoulders under water, legs wide apart, hands on hips, twist round from the waist as far as you can. Do at least four repetitions on both sides, increasing the number as you become more supple.

Stand with your feet apart and knees slightly bent. Hold one or two floats and, stretching your arms out in front, push the float/s round to the right and then to the left, as far as you can go. Keep your feet firm and repeat 16 times.

HYPNO SLIM

Recipes

Our slimmers chose the following recipes because they are
healthy, easy to make and taste delicious. They were supplied
by:

Fresh Fruit & Vegetable Information Bureau
Sea Fish Industry Authority
Handel Communications on behalf of Hellmann's Mayonnaise
Meat and Livestock Commission
Pasta Information Centre
The Cookery Consultancy, Cambridge
British Chicken Information Service
Potato Marketing Board

DIPS, DRINKS AND DRESSINGS

I t's worth making an effort with your dips, drinks and dressings because they will make all the difference to your enjoyment of fresh, raw vegetables. They will help you to start your new lifetime habits. Or at least help you to endure your diet!

FISHY DIP 1
Ingredients
1 small tin mackerel in brine.
75g (3oz) cottage cheese
25g (1 oz) butter
juice 1/2 a lemon
2 finely chopped spring onions
fresh tarragon
pepper

Method
Drain fish and blend with rest of the ingredients until smooth. Chill

FISHY DIP 2
Ingredients
450g (1 lb) smoked mackerel fillets
200g (7 oz) cream cheese
2.5cm (1 inch) piece fresh ginger, peeled and grated
1 green chilli, de-seeded and chopped
2 teaspoons Marmite
1 tablespoons chopped fresh parsley
salt and freshly ground black pepper

Method
Skin the mackerel fillets and break into small pieces. Blend with the other ingredients until smooth. Season to taste and chill. If you want it to be thinner, add lemon juice or plain yoghurt.

CHEESY DIP
Ingredients
cottage cheese
plain yoghurt
spring onions
parsley, finely chopped
salt and freshly ground pepper
The amounts to use depends on your own personal taste.

Method
Blend and chill.

BEAN DIP
Ingredients
125g (4 oz) butter beans (cooked or tinned)
1 clove crushed garlic
1 tablespoon olive oil
salt and freshly ground pepper

Method
Mash the butter beans and mix with garlic, oil and seasoning. Chill.

HUMMUS
Ingredients
125g (4 oz) chick peas, cooked and drained (reserve the water)
1-2 cloves crushed garlic
2 tablespoons lemon juice
2 tablespoons tahini (sesame cream, from health shops)
4 tablespoons olive oil
salt

Method
Blend chick peas with some of the water and the rest of the ingredients.
If you want it thinner, add more cooking water. Chill.

DRINKS

Experiment with any mixture of fruit and vegetables until you find a combination you really enjoy. Garnish with slices of lime, cucumber, orange or lemon peel. (Grate the skin of citrus fruits finely to sprinkle on salads, muesli or cornflakes.) Add herbs - preferably fresh but dried are better than nothing - like sprigs of mint, dill, basil, parsley, tarragon or chives. And top up with chilled sparkling mineral water if you want a longer, thinner drink.

Here are some suggestions:

Orange, grapefruit and lime, plus mineral water
Pineapple, rasberry and apple
Melon and strawberries
Rasberry and apple
Cherry, peach and cucumber
Carrot, apple and courgette
Tomato and carrot
Tomato and orange
Tomato, celery, carrot and apple
Carrot, white cabbage and red pepper

Make your drinks fresh and use as much of the fruit or vegetable as possible.

DRESSINGS

Interesting dressings ARE the difference between monotony and magic meals when you are trying to lose weight. They can turn a dreary salad into a real delight. So forget about fattening mayonnaise and put some life into your salads with these recipes.

FRENCH DRESSING

93

Ingredients
Olive oil
Lemon juice or wine vinegar
French mustard
pinch sugar or quarter teaspoon honey
crushed garlic
fresh herbs
salt and freshly ground black pepper

Method
Combine ingredients in airtight jar.

SOUR CREAM DRESSING
Ingredients
sour cream
tomato juice
lemon juice
paprika

Method
Combine ingredients in proportions to suit yourself.

YOGHURT DRESSING 1
Ingredients
1 tub Greek yoghurt
watercress
grapes
lemon juice
paprika (or curry powder, taste of your choice)

Method
Combine ingredients in proportions to suit yourself.

YOGHURT DRESSING 2
Ingredients
tub natural yoghurt
lemon juice

spring onions
salt and freshly ground pepper

Method
Combine all the ingredients in a blender.

FROMAGE DRESSING
Ingredients
fromage frais
lemon juice
paprika
pinch salt
celery
grapes or orange juice

Method
Combine all the ingredients in a blender.

RAW APPLE, LEMON AND HONEY DRESSING
Ingredients
juice of 1 lemon
4 eating apples, cored and thinly sliced
2 x 5ml (2 tbs) clear honey

Method
Blend apple and lemon juice then mix in honey.

CITRUS DRESSING
Ingredients
juice 2 medium oranges
1 tblsp lemon juice
90ml (3 fl oz) olive oil
salt and pepper

Method
Put the orange and lemon juice in a saucepan and simmer to reduce.
Cool. Pour into a blender, season with salt and pepper, then slowly add

the oil while the machine is running and continue to blend until emulsion is formed. Put the salad ingredients, such as the fennel and mushroom with a selections of lettuces, into a large bowl, pour over the dressing and toss together.

MUSTARD DRESSING
Ingredients
French, whole grain mustard
lemon juice
chopped parsley
water

Method
Combine and chill.

ORANGE CHILLI DRESSING
Ingredients
orange juice
soy sauce to taste
small, fresh green chilli, de-seeded and chopped
1 clove garlic, crushed.

Method
Combine and chill.

SOUP RECIPES

Y ou can make a soup out of almost anything. Cook the ingredients together, steamed, baked or stir fried, throw them in a blender and often, with just a little ingenuity, you have a totally nutritious and satisfying dish. They can be light, to be eaten as a starter, or real rib-stickers, meant to keep you sustained through arduous toil. It is well worth cultivating a way with soups because they can generally be made to be filling and not too fattening at the same time.

POTATO AND BROCCOLI SOUP
Ingredients
1 small onion, peeled and finely chopped
25g butter
450g potatoes, peeled and cut in cubes
25g wholemeal flour
1 pint chicken stock
1/2 pint milk
salt and freshly ground black pepper
150g broccoli, divided into small florets

Method
Fry the onion gently in butter for three minutes. Add the cubed potatoes and fry together with the onion for a further minute. Stir in the flour and gradually stir in the stock and milk. Bring to the boil. Add seasoning to taste and simmer for 10-15 minutes. Add the broccoli and simmer for 4-5 minutes, until the vegetables are just tender. Serve piping hot with crusty wholemeal bread.
Serves 4.

HADDOCK AND SWEETCORN SOUP

Ingredients

1-1/2lb haddock fillets, fresh or defrosted, skinned and cubed
4 sticks celery, sliced
1 pint fish or chicken stock
1/2 pint semi-skimmed milk
10oz can sweetcorn
salt and pepper
2 tbs cornflour (or 1 tbs arrowroot)
2oz peeled prawns (optional)
chopped parsley for garnish

Method

Simmer the celery in the stock until just tender. Add the milk, fish, sweetcorn and seasonings. Simmer gently for 8-10 minutes until the fish is cooked. Take care not to boil vigorously. Blend the cornflour with a little water to make a smooth paste. Stir into the saucepan with the prawns if using. Simmer, stirring occasionally, for 2-3 minutes until the soup has thickened. Serve garnished with chopped parsley.
Serves 6.

Tip. *Try using fresh or defrosted ling or pollack instead of cod or haddock.*

LETTUCE GAZPACHO

Even in winter lettuce is always available, so don't think of gazpacho as a summer-only soup. I think a light soup is the best starter to a meal, and gazpacho is perfect. Beside making sure we are getting the essential vitamins, it helps us to not over-eat the main course.

Ingredients

1 medium onion, peeled and finely chopped
2 cloves garlic, peeled and crushed
3 tbs olive oil
8 tomatoes, quartered
1/2 cucumber, seeded and diced
1/4 pint chicken stock
1 tbs fresh basil, chopped (or 1 tsp dried basil)
salt and freshly ground black pepper

1 iceberg lettuce, finely shredded
parsley or basil to garnish

Method
Fry the onion and garlic gently in the oil for three minutes. Add the red pepper, tomatoes, cucumber, stock, chopped basil, salt and pepper to taste, and bring to the boil. Simmer for five minutes. Add most of the shredded lettuce and simmer for a further three minutes. Blend until smooth. Chill for 4-6 hours. Stir the remaining shredded lettuce into the gazpacho. Ladle into bowls, add an ice cube to each one, and sprinkle with chopped basil or parsley.
Serves 4.

LETTUCE AND TARRAGON SOUP
Ingredients
1/4 iceberg lettuce
1 small onion, finely chopped
25g butter
1 clove garlic, crushed
15g plain flour
1/2 pint chicken stock
3 tbs milk
1/2 tbs chopped fresh tarragon
salt and freshly ground black pepper
few tarragon leaves to garnish

Method
Shred the lettuce finely, keeping back some of the shredded centre leaves for garnish. Fry the onion gently in the butter for 3-4 minutes. Add the garlic and flour, and stir over the heat for one minute. Gradually stir in the stock and milk, and bring to the boil. Add most of the shredded lettuce, the tarragon, salt and pepper to taste. Simmer for 20 minutes. Blend the soup in a liquidiser until smooth. Return to a clean pan and heat through. Add the cream and the reserved shredded lettuce. Serve piping hot, garnished with fresh tarragon and a few more shards of shredded iceberg lettuce.
Serves 2.

LETTUCE VICHYSOISSE

Ingredients

225g leeks, split, cleaned and chopped
225g potatoes, peeled and chopped
1 clove garlic, peeled and crushed
25g butter
175g coarsely chopped iceberg lettuce
900ml (1-1/2 pints) chicken stock
salt and freshly ground black pepper
3 tbs thick natural yoghurt
50g finely shredded iceberg lettuce
iceberg lettuce petals

Method

Fry the chopped leeks, potatoes and garlic gently in the butter for 4-5 minutes. Add the chopped lettuce, chicken stock and salt and pepper to taste. Bring to the boil and simmer gently until the vegetables are just tender. Blend the soup in a liquidiser or food processor until smooth and allow to cool. Whisk the yoghurt into the soup and chill for 3-4 hours. Stir in the shredded lettuce and serve in small shallow soup bowls garnished with lettuce petals.

To make iceberg lettuce petals, choose good-coloured crisp leaves of iceberg, preferably ones that are slightly curly in shape. Using a small fluted pastry cutter, stamp out small round shapes. Put into a bowl of iced water, and drain thoroughly before using.

Serves 4.

PASTA

PASTA WITH SALMON AND WHITE WINE SAUCE
Ingredients
175g (6oz) salmon fillet, skinned
3 tbs white wine
1 tbs chopped fresh dill
1 tbs olive oil
2 tbs low cal creme fraiche or fromage frais
salt and freshly ground black pepper to taste
125g (4oz) tagliatelle verde
1 Knorr pasta cube

Method
Place the salmon in a dish with white wine and dill. Leave to marinate
for 20-30 minutes, turning once. Heat the oil in a pan and poach the
salmon and marinate for 5-7 minutes. Flake the fish and add the creme
fraiche or fromage frais and seasoning to the pan, stirring. Meanwhile,
cook the pasta as usual with the cube.
Serve the sauce with the cooked drained pasta, garnished with sprigs of
dill.
Serves 2-3.

PASTA WITH A HERB SAUCE
Ingredients
125g (4oz) tagliatelle verde
1 Knorr pasta cube
1 tbs olive oil
1/2 tsp lemon rind
1 tbs chopped fresh parsley
1 tbs chopped fresh chives
225g (8oz) can chopped tomatoes, drained

101

salt and freshly ground black pepper to taste
Freshly grated Parmesan cheese

Method
Cook the pasta. Meanwhile, heat the oil and add the lemon rind, herbs
and tomatoes. Heat through for 2-3 minutes. Season the sauce well and
serve immediately with the cooked and drained pasta, sprinkled with
Parmesan cheese.
Serves 2.

SPINACH AND PRAWN HOT PASTA SALAD
Ingredients
200g (7oz) prawns
1 tbs olive oil
juice and grated rind of 1 lime
2 tsp sesame seeds
Salt and freshly ground black pepper to taste
125g (4oz) conchiglie pasta
1 pasta cube
75g (3oz) fresh spinach, washed and torn into bite size pieces
Whole prawns and toasted sesame seeds to garnish

Method
Place the prawns in a bowl. Mix the oil, lime juice and rind, sesame
seeds and seasoning together and pour over the prawns. Leave to
marinate in a cool place for 1 hour. Cook the pasta. Place the cooked
and drained pasta in a large bowl. Add the prawns and marinade and
toss together. Add the spinach and mix well. Serve immediately,
garnished with the whole prawns and toasted sesame seeds.
Serves 3-4.

PASTA PIZZA
Ingredients
100g (40z) short-cut pasta, macaroni, shells, waggon wheels, rollers etc
15g (1/2oz)butter
1 onion, grated
4 eggs

6 tbs semi-skimmed milk
potassium salt and pepper
3 tomatoes, sliced
4 tbs tomato ketchup
75g (3oz) low fat cheese, thinly sliced
6 anchovy fillets (optional)
black olives
oil

Method
Cook pasta. Heat butter in large omelette pan. Add grated onion and
cook gently for 2 minutes. Beat eggs with milk and seasoning and add
the cooked pasta. Pour the egg and pasta mixture into the pan. Cook
over a moderate heat, disturbing the mixture occasionally with a
wooden spoon, so that some of the liquid egg runs to the bottom of the
pan. When the underneath surface of the mixture has set, arrange sliced
tomato on the top and spoon over the ketchup. Top with a generous
layer of cheese. Pop under a moderately hot grill, until the "pizza" rises
and the cheese bubbles. Brush the surface with oil and return to the grill
for a few minutes. Serve immediately, cut into wedges. Garnish with
anchovy fillets and a few black olives.
Serves 4-6.

FISH RECIPES

HERRING KEBABS
Alternate chunks of herring with vegetables. Baste with olive or
sesame oil or a barbecue sauce. Grill for 5-10 minutes and eat alone or
serve with rice or salad.

HERRING BAKE
Dust herring fillets with oatmeal and a little mustard powder. Bake in a
moderate oven until crisp. Serve with carrots and spinach lightly
cooked and mashed potatoes.

KIPPER PATE
Poach kippers for a few minutes in a little water. Allow to cool then
puree flesh with natural yoghurt, garlic and lemon juice. Eat with
crispbread or sticks of celery, carrot etc.

FISH STIR FRY
You can make this with any of your favourite fish. Using only a few
drops of oil, cut fish into strips and toss over medium heat for a few
minutes before adding vegetables. Season with soy sauce.

CHIVE AND MACKEREL PATE
Ingredients
225 g (8oz) hot smoked mackerel fillets, skinned
1 tbs chopped chives
1-2 tsp lemon juice
4 tbs fromage frais or Greek yoghurt
pepper

Method
Place mackerel fillets in a bowl, beat until smooth with a wooden

spoon, or blend. Stir in chives, lemon juice and fromage frais or yoghurt until well blended. Season with pepper and serve with crunchy vegetables and wholemeal toast or spread on water biscuits.

POTATO AND SMOKED MACKEREL SALAD

Ingredients
750g (1-1/2 lb) new potatoes
juice 1 lemon
4 tbs oil
grated rind 1 orange
peeled segments 1 orange
225g (1/2 lb) smoked mackerel fillet, flaked
freshly ground black pepper
1 tsp chopped thyme
sprigs thyme

Method
Cook the new potatoes in boiling salted water in their skins. Drain and slice. Mix the lemon juice and oil with the orange rind and stir into the cooked potatoes while they are still warm. Stir in the orange segments and smoked mackerel, together with salt and pepper and chopped thyme to taste. Spoon onto a shallow serving dish and border with sprigs of fresh thyme.
Serves 4.

KIPPER STIR FRY

Ingredients
225g (1/2 lb) kipper fillets, skinned and sliced
1 tbs sunflower oil
1 clove crushed garlic
1 small onion, thinly sliced
1 red pepper, cored, deseeded and thinly sliced
175 g (6oz) Chinese leaves or white cabbage, shredded
200g (7oz) can sweetcorn, drained
freshly ground black pepper
4 tbs whisky

Method

Heat the oil in a large frying pan or wok. Cook the garlic and onion until soft and transparent. Stir in the peppers and chinese leaves or cabbage and cook for a further 2 minutes. Stir in kippers and cook for 4 minutes, stirring carefully. Add sweetcorn and seasoning. Stir in whisky and flambe. Serve with brown rice.
Serves 4.

SMOKED HADDOCK PATE

Ingredients
350g (12oz) smoked haddock fillet, fresh or defrosted, diced
1/4 pint water
2 tsp lemon juice
4 tbs natural yoghurt or single cream
1 tsp Worcestershire sauce
pepper
cayenne pepper
25-50g (1-2oz) butter, melted

Method

Poach the fish in the water for 5-7 minutes. Drain. Flake the fish or blend. Add the lemon juice, yoghurt or cream, Worcestershire sauce and pepper to taste. Blend until smooth. Spoon into individual dishes, pour over melted butter, chill until set. Serve with toast or crusty bread.
Serves 4.

SPEEDY PLAICE WITH LEEK & POTATO

Ingredients
225g (8oz) plaice fillets, skinned
300g (10oz) can leek and potato soup

Method

Preheat the oven to 190°C/375°F Gas Mark 5
Roll up the plaice fillets with the skinned side inside, arrange in an ovenproof dish. Pour the soup over the fillets. Cover and bake for 35-40 minutes. Serves 4.

WHITE FISH WAFFLES
Ingredients
450g (1 lb) frozen coley or haddock portions
25g (1oz) butter or margarine
salt and pepper
70g (2-1/2oz) frozen sweetcorn
125g (5oz) frozen broccoli florets
90 mls (3 fl oz) single cream or milk
1 egg, beaten
3 potato waffles cut into 4

Method
Preheat oven to 200°C/400°F, Gas Mark 6
Place the fish portions into a lightly greased shallow ovenproof dish.
Season with salt and pepper. Sprinkle over the sweetcorn and broccoli.
Mix together the cream and the egg. Pour over the fish and vegetables.
Top with the waffles. Bake for 35-40 minutes until the fish is cooked.
Serves 4.

CAPTAIN'S FISH BAKE
Ingredients
4 frozen fish steaks in parsley sauce
8oz (225g) frozen stewpack or mixed vegetables
1/2 small onion, chopped
4 slices bread, brown and white
1oz (25g) butter or margarine, softened
1oz (25g) cheese, grated

Method
Preheat oven to 200°C/400°F, Gas Mark 6
Place the unopened bags of fish and sauce into a pan of boiling water.
Bring back to the boil for just 5 minutes. Meanwhile, place the vegetables in the bottom of a shallow ovenproof dish. Transfer the partially cooked fish portions to a plate, cut open the bags and pour the contents on top of the vegetables. Butter the bread, cut into triangles and arrange

over the fish portions, buttered side up. Sprinkle over the grated cheese
and bake for 30-35 minutes until the bread is golden brown and the fish
is cooked.
Serves 4.

*Tip: To adjust the recipe for fresh fillets, arrange four pieces of white
fish fillets in a dish add the vegetables and pour over 1/2 pint (280ml)
parsley sauce. Continue with the recipe.*

LEMON SOLE WITH ALMONDS AND BANANAS
Ingredients
4 x 175g (6oz) lemon sole fillets
25g (1oz) butter or margarine
1 banana, sliced
25g (1oz) flaked almonds
3 tbs lemon juice
salt and pepper
parsley

Method
Cut fillets in half lengthways and fold in two.
Melt butter in a pan and cook fillets for 5-6 minutes, turning once.
Add the bananas, almonds, lemon juice and seasoning. Cover and cook
for 3-4 minutes. Garnish with chopped parsley.
Serves 4.

FISH RECIPES II
(Spicy fish recipes)

COLEY CHILLI POT
Ingredients
675g (1-1/2 lbs) coley fillet, fresh or defrosted, skinned,
or 6 frozen coley portions
15ml (1 tbs) sunflower oil
1 small onion, chopped
1 garlic clove, crushed
1 small green pepper, deseeded and cut into strips
200g (7oz) can chopped tomatoes
400g (14oz) chilli beans
200g (7oz) baked beans
salt and pepper

Method
Heat the oil in a large shallow pan. Cook the onions, garlic and green
pepper for 1-2 minutes. Stir in the chopped tomatoes, chilli beans and
baked beans. Bring to the boil, stirring occasionally, reducing the heat.
Cut the fish into six portions and add to the pan. Cover and simmer for
10-15 minutes (15-20 if frozen). Season to taste. Serve with pasta and a
green salad.
Serves 6.

FISH TIKKA
Ingredients
200g (8oz) cod steaks
1/4 pint natural yoghurt
garlic
1/2 tsp ground chilli
1 tsp garam masala

1/2 tsp ground ginger
1 tbs lemon juice
salt and pepper
2 drops red food colouring

Method
Place fish in a shallow dish. Mix together remaining ingredients in a
small bowl. Pour over the cod steaks. Cover and refrigerate for 2-4
hours. Grill for 10-15 minutes.
Serves 2.

PRAWN MADRAS
Ingredients
2lbs (900g) small, cooked, peeled, warm water prawns, fresh or defrosted
1oz (25g) butter
1 large onion, sliced
2 garlic cloves, crushed
2 tbs (30ml) curry powder
salt and pepper
2 tbs (30ml) lemon juice
4 tbs (60ml) fish or chicken stock
2 tbs (30ml) tomato puree
coriander or parsley leaves to garnish

Method
Heat butter and oil in a large frying pan. Cook the onions and garlic
until soft. Stir in the curry powder, seasoning and lemon juice, cook for
a further 2 minutes. Stir in stock and tomato puree, simmer for 5
minutes. Add prawns and cook for a further 2 minutes, until piping hot.
Serve with rice.
Serves 4.

SEAFISH CREOLE
Ingredients
1 to 1-1/2lbs (450-675g) cod or ling fillets, fresh or defrosted, skinned
and cubed

Spicy Fish

1 tbs (15ml) oil
1 clove garlic, crushed
1 onion, sliced
1" (2.5cm) piece root ginger, peeled and finely chopped
2 tsp (10ml) ground coriander
1 tsp (5ml) turmeric
1 tsp (5ml) ground cumin
1 tsp (5ml) paprika
1 tbs (15ml) flour
1/4 pint (140ml) fish or vegetable stock
7oz (200g) can tomatoes
8oz (225g) can pineapple cubes in natural juice
1 bay leaf
salt and pepper

Method
Heat the oil in a large pan, cook the garlic, onion and ginger until onion is soft. Stir in the spices and flour, cook for about 1 minute. Gradually stir in the stock, tomatoes and pineapple together with the juice. Bring to the boil add the bayleaf and seasoning, simmer uncovered for about 10 minutes. Add the fish and simmer for a further 7-10 minutes, remove the bayleaf. Serve with rice and a crisp salad.
Serves 4-6.

STIR-FRIED CRAB
Ingredients
1lb (450g) crabmeat, fresh or defrosted
1 tbs (15ml) oil
4 sticks celery, sliced
1 large red pepper, deseeded and sliced lengthways
2oz (50g) sliced mushrooms
2-3 tsp (10-15ml) light soya sauce
black pepper
lettuce leaves for serving

Method
Heat the oil in a wok or large, shallow frying pan. Add all the vegeta-

bles and toss for 2-3 minutes. Add the crabmeat, soy sauce and black pepper and toss for another 2-3 minutes until heated through. Serve on lettuce leaves.
Serves 4.

SMOKY FISH FRICASSEE

Ingredients
450g (1 lb) smoked cod, haddock or whiting fillets, skinned and cubed
225g (8oz) frozen, mixed vegetables
500g (18oz) can new potatoes, drained and quartered OR
450g small new potatoes, scrubbed, quartered and cooked
3-4 drops Tabasco sauce
3 tbs single cream
1 tbs chopped parsley

Method
Place vegetables in a large shallow pan with 3 tablespoons of water. Cover and cook for one minute. Stir in the potatoes and cook for a further 3-4 minutes. Carefully stir in fish and add Tabasco. Cover and simmer for 5 minutes. Pour over the cream, add the parsley, cook uncovered until hot.
Serves 4.

SPICY CURRY COLEY

Ingredients
450g (1 lb) coley or pollack fillets, fresh or defrosted, skinned and cubed
15ml (1 tbs) sunflower oil
1 small onion, chopped
2 sticks celery, chopped
5-10ml (1-2 tsp) curry powder
197g (7oz) can chopped tomatoes
400g (14oz) can baked beans
1 red apple, cored and diced
salt and pepper

Spicy Fish

Method

Heat the oil in a large pan. Cook the onion and celery for 1-2 minutes or until soft. Stir in the curry powder, tomatoes, baked beans and apples. Bring to the boil reduce the heat and stir in the fish. Simmer gently for 10-12 minutes. Season to taste.
Serves 4.

PIZZA

EASY PEASY PIZZA
Ingredients
1 smallish French baguette or two slices wholemeal bread
1 chopped onion
1 small can tomatoes, drained (no sugar)
1 small can sardines in brine, drained
1 tbs tomato puree
1 tsp oil
garlic
herbs

Method
Fry onion and garlic in the oil. Add tomatoes, puree and herbs. Simmer for a few minutes then add sardines. Meanwhile toast bread gently and when just tinged brown, add pizza topping. Grill to your liking
Serves 2..

CHICKEN RECIPES

CHICKEN CAJUN STYLE
Ingredients
16 chicken wings
4 tsp paprika
2 tsp ground coriander
1 tsp celery salt
1 tsp ground cumin
1/2 tsp cayenne
1/2 tsp salt
1 tbs oil
2 tbs red wine vinegar
extra oil for brushing

Method
Wash and dry the chicken wings, removing wing tips.
Mix together the paprika, coriander, celery salt, cumin, cayenne, salt,
oil and vinegar. Rub this mixture into the wings and set aside, in the
refrigerator, for at least one hour for the flavours to permeate. Cook the
wings over a barbeque grill, brushing with oil, for about 15 minutes,
turning regularly.
Serves 4.

CHINESE WRAPPED CHICKEN
Ingredients
4 boneless, skinless chicken breasts
1 clove garlic, chopped
1 cm (1/2 in) cube ginger, peeled and finely chopped
1 tbs soy sauce
2 tbs dry sherry

pinch five-spice powder
8 large Chinese leaves
1 large carrot, cut into thin strips
40g shredded mange tout
4 spring onions, sliced

Method
Put the chicken breasts into a shallow dish. Mix together the garlic,
ginger, soy sauce, sherry and five-spice powder, pour over the chicken
and leave to marinate in the refrigerator.
Meanwhile, to soften the chinese leaves, either steam for 1 minute or
plunge into a large pan of boiling water for 1 minute, remove and cool.
To assemble the chicken parcels, place two leaves, slightly overlapping
on a flat surface. Place a quarter of the vegetable mixture in the centre
and top with a chicken breast. Spoon over a little of the marinade then
fold the leaves over to make a parcel, place in a steamer with the ends
of the leaves underneath so the parcel doesn't come undone. Repeat
with the rest of the ingredients and steam the parcels until chicken is
cooked (approx half an hour). Serve with rice.
Serves 4.

HONEYED CHICKEN SALAD
Ingredients
4 boned chicken breasts, skinned
2 sprigs parsley
a few celery leaves
salt and pepper

Marinade
2 tbs olive oil
1 tbs clear honey
4 tbs orange juice
1 tsp coriander seeds, slightly crushed
1 large head chicory
2 handfuls curly endive
2 oranges, peeled and segmented
3 tbs plain yoghurt

1 small onion, thinly sliced

Method
To cook the chicken breasts, either place in a frying pan with the parsley, celery leaves and seasoning, add 600ml (1 pint) water and poach for 10 minutes; or place each breast in a piece of foil, add the parsley and celery, leaves and seasoning, then wrap up and steam for 20-30 minutes until tender. Let them cool.
Mix together the ingredients for the marinade. Slice the chicken breasts and place in a shallow dish, pour over the marinade, cover and refrigerate for at least 2 hours. To serve, chop the chicory and arrange on serving plates with the endive. Place sliced chicken on top with the orange segments. Mix the marinade with the yoghurt and spoon over. Garnish with onion rings.
Serves 4.

SWEET & SOUR DRUMSTICKS
Ingredients
8 chicken drumsticks
4 tbs red wine vinegar
2 tbs tomato puree
2 tbs soy sauce
2 tbs clear honey
1 tbs Worcestershire sauce
2 cloves garlic
good pinch cayenne
salt and pepper

Method
Put the chicken drumsticks into a container, mix together all the other ingredients and pour over the chicken. Allow to marinade in the refrigerator for at least 1 hour or, if possible, overnight.
Prepare the barbecue and cook the drumsticks for about 20 minutes, brushing with the marinade during cooking and turning thoroughly.
Serves 4.

OATY CHICKEN PIECES

Ingredients
4 chicken quarters
25g (1oz) rolled oats
1 tbs chopped fresh rosemary
salt and ground black pepper
1 egg white
150g (6oz) natural low fat fromage frais
2 tsp wholegrain mustard
sprigs of rosemary for garnish

Method
Remove skin from the chicken and pre-heat the oven
Mix together the oats, rosemary, salt and pepper. Brush each piece of
chicken evenly with egg white, then coat in the oat mixture. Place on a
baking sheet and bake for about 40 minutes or until the chicken juices
run clear when pierced. Mix together the fromage frais and mustard,
season to taste then serve with the chicken, hot or cold, garnished with
rosemary.
Serves 4.

LAMB RECIPES

TURKISH CUCUMBER, YOGHURT AND LAMB SALAD
Ingredients
1 cucumber, sliced
200ml (7 fl oz) tub yoghurt
2 cloves garlic, crushed
freshly ground black pepper
2 tbs chopped fresh mint
350g (12oz) cooked lamb, (it should be pink) cut into strips
shredded Cos, Webbs or Iceberg lettuce
fresh mint
12 black olives

Method
Put the cucumber slices into a colander and sprinkle generously with
salt. Leave to drain for 30 minutes. Mix the well-drained cucumber with
the yoghurt, garlic, salt and pepper to taste and chopped fresh mint. Stir
in the lamb. Arrange on a bed of lettuce and garnish with sprigs of mint
and black olives.
Serves 4.

LAMB CASSEROLE WITH CUMIN
Ingredients
675g (1-1/2lb) lamb cut into one inch cubes
2 onions, sliced
4 carrots, in thin strips
2 sticks celery, in thin strips
1/2 pint (300ml) tomato juice
2 x 5ml (2 tsp) ground cumin
1 clove garlic, crushed
salt and pepper

100g (4oz) mushrooms, sliced
50g (2oz) frozen peas

Method
Place the cubed lamb, onions, carrots and celery in a casserole. Mix the
tomato juice, ground cumin, garlic and seasoning and pour over the
lamb and vegetables. Cover and cook in the oven for one hour. Add the
mushrooms and frozen peas and cook for a further 30 minutes.
Serves 4.

LAMB RISOTTO WITH LEMON AND MINT
Ingredients
225g (8oz) lamb neck fillet, or leg steaks cut into cubes
1 tsp oil
1 clove crushed garlic
100g (4oz) easy cook, long grain white rice
1 lemon, grated rind and juice
300ml (1/2 pint) stock
50g (2oz) button mushrooms, quartered
5 spring onions, sliced
2 tbs fresh mint, chopped

Method
Heat the oil in a saucepan. Add the lamb and garlic and cook until
browned. Add the rice and cook for 1-2 minutes. Stir in the lemon and
juice, stock and seasoning. Cover and cook for 20 minutes, stirring
occasionally. Add mushrooms and spring onions. Cover and cook for a
further five minutes or until the liquid has been absorbed and the rice
cooked. Stir in the mint and serve immediately.
Serves 2.

PORK RECIPES

PORK WITH LEEKS AND LENTILS

Ingredients:
4 lean pork steaks or chops
15ml (1 tbs) vegetable oil
1 clove garlic, crushed
5ml (1 tsp) paprika
15ml (1 tbs) tomato puree
150ml (1/4pt) white wine
397g (14oz) can tomatoes, chopped
75g (3oz) red lentils
450g (1lb) leeks, sliced
5ml (1 tsp) dried mixed herbs
Salt and black pepper
fresh parsley, chopped

Method
Heat oil in a large pan, add steaks or chops and garlic, season well.
Cook on each side until browned. Set aside. To the pan, add the paprika
and tomato puree, stir in wine and tomatoes. Bring to the boil, add
lentils. Place leeks in the bottom of a large ovenproof dish, place steaks
or chops on top and pour over tomato mixture. Cover and cook for
approximately 50-60 minutes or until meat is tender and lentils are
cooked. Stir occasionally. Sprinkle with parsley. Serve with new
potatoes and a side salad.
Serves 4.

FRUIT KEBABS

Ingredients
2 eating apples, preferably with pretty skins
2 conference pears, not too ripe

juice of 1 lemon
8 rashers streaky bacon
2 large pork escalopes, pounded until quite thin
oil
salt and freshly ground black pepper
50g (2oz) fresh breadcrumbs
finely grated rind 1/2 lemon
1 spring onion, very finely chopped
1 tbs chopped fresh basil
sprigs fresh basil to garnish

Method

Halve the apples and pears and remove the cores, then cut in half once
again. Toss prepared fruits in lemon juice. Stretch the bacon rashers
slightly with the back of a knife. Cut each pork escalope into four long,
wide strips. Roll each piece of apple up in a rasher of bacon. Roll each
section of pear up in a strip of pork. Thread alternately onto four small
kebab skewers. Brush with oil and season. Grill for 8-10 minutes.
Meanwhile melt the butter and fry the breadcrumbs until crisp and
golden. Stir in the lemon rind, spring onion and chopped basil. Arrange the kebabs on a serving dish, sprinkle with the flavoured crumbs
and garnish with sprigs of basil.
Serves 4.

BEEF RECIPES

STIR FRY WITH ORANGE AND CHILLI
Ingredients
450g (1 lb) beef, cut into thin strips
2 tsp dark soy sauce
2 tsp sherry
2 tsp cornflour
1 tsp sesame oil
1/2 inch cube root ginger, peeled and grated
1 tbs oil
1 tsp peppercorns, crushed
1/2 tsp brown sugar
1/2 tsp dried red chillies, chopped
1 orange, grated rind and juice

Method
Mix the marinade ingredients together. Add the meat and make sure it
all gets coated. Cover and put in refrigerator for 15 minutes. Heat oil
in a wok and stir fry the meat for 3-4 minutes. Add the remaining
ingredients and cook for a further 2-3 minutes. Serve immediately with
noodles or rice. Serves 4.

MINCE, LEEK & POTATO BAKE
Ingredients
450g (1 lb) minced beef
1 chopped onion
1 crushed clove garlic
2 tbs tomato ketchup
400 g tin tomatoes
1 tbs mixed herbs
50g split red lentil

1/4 pint stock
salt and black pepper
Topping
675 g (1-1/2 lb) potatoes, peeled and sliced
2 large leeks, trimmed and sliced
25 g (1oz) grated Cheddar cheese

Method
Dry fry the mince, onion and garlic until browned. Add tomato
ketchup, herbs, lentils, stock and seasoning. Simmer, uncovered for 15
minutes. Meanwhile, boil potatoes and leeks in a pan of lightly salted
water for 5 minutes and drain. Place a layer of mince in the bottom of
an ovenproof dish then a layer of leeks and potatoes. Repeat. Sprinkle
with the cheese. Cook in a pre-heated oven until golden. Serve with a
selection of green vegetables. Serves 4.

OFFAL RECIPES

BROWN OWL'S ITALIAN LIVER
(Recipe supplied by Anne Jones)
Ingredients
12oz lamb's liver
1oz flour
salt and pepper
1-1/2oz butter
1 lb onions
1/4 pint beef stock
1/2 pint milk
2 level tbs tomato puree
1 clove chopped garlic
1/4 tsp mixed herbs

Method
Cut liver into small pieces and coat in seasoned flour. Melt butter in a
frying pan and add liver. Brown on both sides then remove from the
pan.
In the remaining butter, fry the onions until tender. Gradually stir in the
stock, milk, tomato puree, garlic and herbs. Bring the sauce to the boil,
stirring continuously. Add the liver to the sauce. Cover pan and cook
gently for 10-15 minutes until liver is tender.
Serves 3.

PAPRIKA LIVER
Ingredients
450 g (1 lb) calf's or lamb's liver
1-1/2 tbs paprika

flour
olive oil
salt
chopped parsley

Method
Wash the liver and cut into small pieces. Drain and sprinkle with most
of the paprika then roll in flour. Fry in oil, stirring and turning until the
pieces are well browned but they should be pink and juicy inside.
Remove, drain and sprinkle with salt. Mix the remaining paprika with
the oil in the pan and dribble over the liver. Serve garnished with
chopped parsley.
Serves 4.

LAMB'S LIVER WITH ORANGE
Ingredients
450 g (1 lb) lamb's liver
juice and finely grated rind of 1 orange
150 g (6 oz) chopped onions
olive oil
seasoning

Method
Remove all sinews from liver and marinate in orange juice, zest and
freshly ground pepper for at least four hours. Fry the onion and remove
from pan. Turn up the heat and flash fry the liver to seal it, return
onions and pour on marinade. Add salt and transfer to casserole. Bake
in a moderate oven for 15 minutes. Serves 4.

LIVER IN VINEGAR
Ingredients
450 g (1 lb) calf's or lamb's liver
150 g (6 oz) dry wholemeal breadcrumbs
1/4 pint white wine vinegar
oil
chopped parsley
salt and pepper

Method
Fry the breadcrumbs and crushed garlic in hot oil, add vinegar and seasoning and bring to the boil. Poach the slices of liver making sure they are not over-cooked. Serve with chopped parsley.
Serves 4.

LIVER AND BACON IN TOMATO SAUCE
Ingredients
450g (1 lb) lamb's liver, sliced
50g (2oz) plain flour, seasoned with black pepper
4 rashers of lean, greenback bacon, no fat
can tomatoes
1 onion, sliced
5ml (1 tsp) sunflower oil
5ml (1 tsp) arrowroot
water

Method
Heat the oil and gently fry onions. Remove with slotted spoon and place in a casserole. Coat liver with seasoned flour and fry until lightly browned. Remove and place on top of onions in casserole. Place bacon rashers on top of the liver and add the tomatoes. Cook for 30 minutes. Make arrowroot into a paste and add to casserole to thicken gravy.
Serves 4.

KIDNEYS TURBIGO
Ingredients
4 lambs kidneys, skinned and cut in half
150g (6oz) low fat pork chipolata sausages
1 tbs corn or sunflower oil
12 button onions
100g (4oz) mushrooms, quartered if large
2 tsp plain flour
2 tbs dry sherry
150ml (1/4 pint) stock
salt and pepper

chopped parsley

Method
Heat the oil in frying pan and brown kidneys. Remove from the pan, then add and brown the chipolatas. Remove chipolatas, add onions and mushrooms and cook these for 2-3 minutes. Stir in the flour, sherry, stock and seasoning. Bring to the boil. Cut the chipolatas in half and return to pan with kidneys. Cover and simmer for 20-25 minutes. Sprinkle with chopped parsley.
Serves 2.

KIDNEYS IN TOMATO SAUCE
Ingredients
2 kidneys per person
2 onions, sliced
4 tomatoes, skinned and chopped (or four tinned, peeled tomatoes)
tomato puree
3 tbs olive oil
crushed garlic
3 tbs vinegar
salt and pepper

Method
Fry the onions and garlic in oil. Wash the kidneys and remove outer skin and fat. Drain and cut in half. Add them to the pan and fry briefly before adding the tomatoes, puree, vinegar and seasoning. Cook for 15-20 minutes.

VEGETABLE RECIPES

COPPER'S WOKPOT
This is one of Andrew's specials
Ingredients
8 oz diced raw turkey
packet of mixed pearl barley/lentils/dried peas
onions
carrots
leeks
garlic
cardamom pods
fresh chillies (if the children aren't eating it)
oil
mixed herbs
soy sauce
wine vinegar
salt and pepper

Method
Soak pulses overnight in cold water and cook for 30 minutes. Heat oil
in wok (just enough to moisten) and stir fry onions, garlic and fresh
chillies. Add turkey, vegetables, cardamom, soy sauce and wine
vinegar, herbs and seasoning. Cook 10 minutes. Serves 3-4.

AUTUMN VEGETABLE CASSEROLE
Ingredients
300g (10oz) turnips
300g (10oz) carrots
300g (10oz) swede
2 sticks celery, sliced
175g (7oz) shallots, peeled

2 medium leeks, thickly sliced
2 tbs oil
1/2 pint chicken stock
400g (14oz) can tomatoes
pinch mixed herbs
salt and freshly ground black pepper
2 tsp cornflour

Topping
125g (5oz) wholemeal plain flour
125g (5oz) plain flour
1/2 tsp salt
2 tsp baking powder
50g (2oz) margarine
1/2 tsp dried sage
1 tbs chopped parsley
50g (2oz) Cheddar cheese, finely grated
150 ml (1/4 pint) plain yoghurt
2 tbs milk

Method
Peel turnip, carrots and swede and cut into chunks. Cook in oil until
beginning to brown. Turn into a casserole dish and pour over the stock,
tomatoes and season with herbs, salt and pepper. Cover and cook for 30
minutes. Blend the cornflour with water, remove casserole and stir into
vegetables. Cover and cook for a further 10 minutes. Meanwhile,
make the topping by mixing the flours and baking powder and rubbing
in the margarine. Add sage, parsley and cheese then mix to a soft
dough with the yoghurt and milk. Lightly knead the dough until
smooth then roll out about 1/2 inch thick. Cut out rounds and put them
on top of vegetables, slightly overlapping. Brush with a little milk. Put
the uncovered dish back in the oven and cook for a further 20 minutes
until the topping is risen and golden. Serves 6.

BEAN PIE
This is one of Janice's Farmer's Fare standbys which looks a bit like
chilli con carne but there's no meat. Janis doesn't measure the ingredi-

ents because it depends what she's got. Sounds like my kind of cook.

Ingredients

Tin drained red kidney beans

Tinned or fresh tomatoes

Mushrooms

Onions

Mashed potato

Tomato puree

Chilli paste to taste

Herbs, salt and pepper

Method

Put all the other ingredients in a casserole and spread the mashed potato on top. Bake until golden. Serves 4-8, depending on what you put in!

BROWN OWL VEGETABLE BAKE

This one is Anne's own recipes

Ingredients

Carrots, leeks, cabbage, onion, peas, green beans

6oz potato, cooked

4oz mushrooms

3 tbs stuffing mix

1 teaspoon mixed herbs

cup of breadcrumbs

1/2 pint vegetable stock

Method

Chop and cook vegetables and place in ovenproof dish. Sprinkle with mixed herbs and stuffing mixture between layers. Slice mushrooms and place over the other vegetables. Slice the precooked potatoes, carefully lay across the top of the dish and sprinkle with breadcrumbs. Pour over the vegetable stock.

Bake in 180°C, 375°F, Gas Mark 5 oven for 20 minutes until piping hot or reheat in microwave for seven minutes and place under hot grill for 5 minutes to crisp up top.

Serves 4.

EGG & VEGETABLE SAUTE
Ingredients
5ml (1 tsp) vegetable oil
4 eggs, size 3, beaten
1 medium onion, roughly chopped
1 clove garlic, crushed
525g (1-1/4lbs) potatoes, peeled, coarsely grated, rinsed and dried
1 medium red pepper, deseeded and cut into strips
125g (5oz) mushrooms, halved
4 tomatoes, sliced
125g (5oz) baby sweetcorns, halved
125g (5oz) mange tout, topped and tailed
125g (5oz) broccoli, broken into small florets
15ml (1 tbs) tomato puree
30ml (2 tbs) tomato ketchup
45ml (3 tbs) light soy sauce
freshly ground black pepper, garnish with lemon wedges

Method
Heat the oil in a wok or large frying pan, add the beaten egg and cook
as an omelette for 2 minutes. Remove to a plate. Fry the onion and
garlic together in the same pan for 1 minute. Add the potato and stir fry
for 5 minutes. Add the remaining vegetables and fry, stirring occasionally for a further 15-20 minutes until the potato is just cooked. Roughly
chop the omelette and add to the vegetable mixture. Stir in the tomato
puree, tomato ketchup, soy sauce and cook for a further five minutes.
Season well. Garnish and serve with a green vegetable.
Serves 4.

GRILLED SUMMER VEGETABLE WITH PESTO SAUCE
Ingredients
2 small aubergines
4 medium courgettes
1 yellow pepper
1 red pepper
225g (8oz) large cap mushrooms
6 tbs olive oil

1 tbs red wine vinegar
1 clove garlic
1/2 tsp dried oregano
1/2 tsp dried thyme
salt and pepper
Pesto Sauce:
25g (1oz) fresh basil leaves
2 cloves garlic
25g (1oz) pine nuts
4 tbs virgin olive oil
25g (1oz) freshly grated Parmesan cheese

Method
Cut the aubergines into slices about 1/4 inch thick, sprinkle with salt
and place between two large plates with a weight on top until bitter
juice comes out. Dab away with kitchen paper. Cut the courgettes
diagonally about half inch thick and put into large dish with aubergines.
Cut the peppers into strips an add with the trimmed mushrooms. Mix
together the oil, vinegar, garlic and herbs and seasoning. Pour over the
vegetables coating them evenly. Cover the dish and refrigerate for 2
hours or overnight.
To make the pesto, wash and dry the basil leaves, put into a blender or
food processor with garlic, pine nuts and oil and work until smooth.
Turn into a bowl and beat in the Parmesan cheese, then transfer to
serving dish.
Grill vegetables until tender, basting them with the marinade during
cooking. Arrange the vegetables on a warm plate and serve with the
pesto sauce.

Serves 2-3.

PULSE RECIPES

LENTIL BAKE
Ingredients
1 onion
1 tbs olive oil (or a little vegetable stock)
6oz split red lentils
1 lb fennel or celery
3/4 pint stock
1 bay leaf
juice of a lemon
salt, pepper
dried wholemeal breadcrumbs
1 tsp grated cheese

Method
Soften onions and add washed lentils. Cook until soft and liquidise with lemon juice, salt and pepper. Slice and cook *al denté* the fennel or celery and place in the bottom of a greased ovenproof dish. Pour the lentil mixture over and sprinkle with crumbs and cheese. Bake for 30 minutes, finishing off under the grill to give it a golden glow. Serves 2.

LENTILS AND PASTA
Ingredients
200g brown lentils, cooked
200g tomatoes, peeled and chopped
100g mushrooms
2 medium-sized onions
2 carrots
celery
cooking apples
1 clove crushed garlic

tomato puree
olive oil
stock
lemon juice
oregano
salt and pepper

Method
Chop the vegetables and fry in oil until soft. Mix in all remaining
ingredients and simmer, covered, for approximately 45 minutes. serve
with wholewheat pasta and sprinkle with parmesan cheese.

LENTIL PIE
Ingredients
200g (6oz) lentils
1 large onion
1 clove crushed garlic
chopped celery
diced carrot
chopped mushrooms
1 tbs tomato puree
marjoram, thyme, salt and pepper
olive oil or small amount of vegetable stock
800g mashed potato
sprinkle of parmesan or small amount of margarine

Method
Soak, drain, rinse lentils and cook lentils until tender. Fry vegetables in
oil or stock until tender, then add to lentils. Mix in tomato puree, herbs,
salt and pepper and spoon into a greased ovenproof dish. Cover with
mashed potato and dot with margarine or sprinkle with parmesan and
bake in a moderate oven until golden. Serves 4-6.

LENTIL SPAGHETTI BOLOGNAISE
Ingredients
200g (60z) lentils
120g mushrooms

3 carrots
4 sticks celery
2 onions
1 cooking apple
1 clove crushed garlic
tomato puree to taste
olive oil
1 pint stock
1/2 pint cider
juice of a lemon
1 tsp oregano
salt and freshly ground black pepper

Method
Soak lentils in water with bay leaf overnight then cook until tender. Stir fry chopped vegetables in oil. Add all the remaining ingredients and simmer, covered, for 30 minutes or so. Serve with wholewheat spaghetti and sprinkle with parmesan.
Serves 4-6.

COTTAGE PIE
Ingredients
250g lentils soaked and cooked until tender (retain water)
500g mashed potato
250g variety of vegetables, grated (carrot, parsnip, swede, turnip)
small cauliflower
2 tbs tomato puree
2 tbs yeast extract
2 tbs sunflower oil
salt and pepper

Method
Stir fry vegetables in oil then add lentils, stirring to combine the mixture before transferring to a casserole. Mix the tomato puree, yeast extract and the water in which the lentils were cooked, season with salt and pepper and pour into casserole. Top with mashed potato and dot with margarine. Bake for 30 minutes in a medium oven. Serve with

slightly steamed green leafy vegetables like spinach or cabbage, or
peas. Serves 4-6.

HARICOT BEAN PUREE

A bean puree is very easy to make and can be a useful addition to
vegetable soups to give them body, or eaten as a starter with warm pitta
bread.

Ingredients

250g haricot beans (or red kidney beans, or chick peas)
4 tbs olive oil
juice of 1 or 2 lemons
any fresh herb (optional)
salt and freshly ground black pepper.

Method

Soak the beans overnight in water with a bay leaf, then cook them until
tender. Drain, add the olive oil, lemon juice, seasoning and optional
fresh herb and blend. Serves 2-4.

SALAD RECIPES

COTTAGE CHEESE AND PRAWN SALAD
Ingredients
175g cottage cheese
175g peeled prawns
450g new potatoes, scrubbed, quartered, cooked and cooled
1/4 red cabbage, finely shredded
1/4 cucumber, diced
salt and freshly ground black pepper
4 tbs low calorie mayonnaise
1 tsp paprika
lemon quarters and prawns to garnish

Method
Mix all the ingredients except the mayonnaise together in a large bowl.
Season well. Place in a serving dish, spoon over mayonnaise and
sprinkle with paprika. Garnish and serve on a bed of cucumber, with
biscuits.
Serves 4.

APPLE AND NUT SALAD
Ingredients
1 apple per person, chopped
1 stick celery per person, chopped
1 bunch spring onions, sliced
1 cucumber, diced
natural peanuts
lemon juice

Method
Sprinkle lemon juice on apples. Mix ingredients together and toss in a French dressing.

JAPANESE-STYLE CUCUMBER AND CARROT SALAD
Ingredients
1 large cucumber
1 small carrot
1 tbs dehulled sesame seeds
2 tbs soy sauce
2 dsp distilled white vinegar

Method
Peel the cucumber and cut it wafer-thin. Peel the carrot and cut in the same way. Brown the sesame seeds on a tray under the grill. (They are ready when they start popping.) Pour the soy sauce and vinegar over the cucumber and carrot and mix thoroughly. Sprinkle on sesame seeds and mix again.
Serves 2.

PASTA SALAD
Ingredients
200g dried pasta shapes
1 chopped red pepper
1 small can sweetcorn
sunflower oil
lemon juice to taste
crushed garlic to taste
chopped parsley

Method
Cook pasta, drain and rinse. Mix in pepper and sweetcorn. Mix other ingredients together and pour over the pasta. Toss to coat thoroughly.

TROPICAL PASTA SALAD
Ingredients
125g (5oz) pasta shells
1 pasta stock cube
1 red apple, skin on, chopped and tossed in lemon juice
1 tbs lime juice
75g melon balls
50g cashew nuts
1 banana, sliced
1 tbs mayonnaise
2 tbs watercress, trimmed

Method
Cook the pasta in stock prepared with the stock cube, and allow to cool.
Combine all other ingredients and mix into the pasta. Serve chilled,
garnished with sprigs of watercress.
Serves 3-4.

PUDDING RECIPES

CHOCOLATE MOUSSE
Ingredients
14oz (400g) dark chocolate
8 eggs
3 tbs rum
1 orange
4 tsp ground coffee
pinch of salt

Method
Make half a cup of coffee and put it, with the rum and chocolate broken into pieces, into the top of a double boiler and melt until the mixture is smooth. Lightly whisk the yolks and add to the chocolate mixture along with half the grated orange peel. Beat the egg whites with a pinch of salt until stiff and fold in. Pour into a large bowl or individual pots, sprinkle with the rest of the orange zest, and refrigerate for at least six hours. Serves 6.

FRUIT MONT BLANC
Ingredients
200g (7oz) eating apples, thinly sliced
grated rind of a medium orange
orange slices
white of one egg
water (or you can add orange juice)

Method
Put the apple and orange rind in a saucepan with the water. Cook gently until the apple is soft and make sure it doesn't dry up. Puree in a blender. Whisk the egg white until stiff and fold into the apple mixture.

Arrange it on top of orange slices and chill.
Serves 2.

BLACK GRAPE CURD CAKE

(This one is only allowed when you have reached your target. It's
healthy but very naughty.)

Ingredients

225g (8oz) black grapes, halved and deseeded
1 lemon rind, finely grated
3 tsp (15ml) lemon juice
50g (2oz) caster sugar
125g (5oz) curd cheese
3 eggs, size 2, separated
225g (1/2lb) potatoes, peeled, cooked, sieved and cooled
5ml (1 tsp) baking powder
icing sugar to dust
decoration: frosted grapes

Method

Pre-heat oven to 180°C, 350°F, Gas Mark 4.
Sprinkle grapes with lemon juice and 1 tablespoon of caster sugar and
set aside. Mix the cheese with the remaining sugar then beat in the egg
yokes, one at a time, and the lemon rind. Add the potato and baking
powder and beat into the mixture. Whisk egg whites until stiff. Beat 3
tablespoons of egg white into the cheese mixture, then carefully fold in
the remainder together with the grape halves. Pour the mixture into an
ovenproof dish and bake for 40-45 minutes or until firm to the touch.
Sprinkle with icing sugar and serve hot or cold with natural yoghurt or
no fat ice cream.
Serves 6.

COCOA AND BLACK CHERRY CAKE

Ingredients

225g (8 oz) potatoes, peeled, cooked, sieved and cooled
25g (1oz) cocoa powder, sieved
50g (2oz) ground almonds
15ml (1 tbs) water

75g (3oz) caster sugar
4 eggs, size 2, separated
Topping
225g (8oz) low fat Greek yoghurt
30 ml (2 dsp) black cherry conserve

Method
Place the potato in a bowl and mix with the cocoa, almonds and water
until a paste is formed. Place the sugar and egg yolks in a large bowl
and stand over a pan of hot water. Whisk until pale, thick and creamy.
Add to the potato mixture and whisk quickly for 15 seconds until
blended. Whisk the egg whites until stiff. With a metal spoon, fold into
the potato mixture and whisk for a further 10 seconds until the mixture
is blended and smooth. Pour into a greased, lined 18 cm (7") square
baking tin and bake in a 190°C, 375°F, Gas Mark 5 oven for 20-25
minutes until firm to the touch. Allow to cool. Spread the cake with
Greek yoghurt and using a teaspoon, dot the conserve at regular
intervals over the yoghurt. With a skewer, gradually draw lines through
the conserve creating a swirl effect. Cut into squares and serve.
Serves 9.

FRUIT AND SPICE LOAF
Ingredients
125g (5oz) polyunsaturated margarine
125g (5oz) molasses sugar
2 eggs, size 3 beaten
75g (3oz) dates, stoned and chopped
50g (2oz) sultanas
50g (2oz) dried apricots, chopped
50g (2oz) walnuts, roughly chopped
5ml (1 tsp) ground ginger
5ml (1 tsp) mixed spice
175g (7oz) potatoes, peeled, grated coarsely, rinsed and dried
75g (3oz) self-raising flour
75g (3oz) wholemeal flour
5ml (1 tbs) baking powder

Method
Line and lightly grease a 900g (2 lb) loaf tin. Cream the margarine and
sugar together until well blended. Gradually beat in the eggs. Add the
fruit, nuts, spices and potato. Mix thoroughly. Fold in the flours and
baking powder. Spoon into the tin, cover with a piece of greaseproof
paper and bake in a 180°C, 375°F, Gas Mark 5 oven for 45 minutes or
until a skewer, when inserted into the centre, comes out clean. Turn out
onto a cooling rack and allow to cool completely before slicing. Serve
on its own or warm with plain low fat yoghurt.
Serves 10.

NOT NAUGHTY ICE CREAM
Ingredients
6 ripe bananas, peeled, sliced and frozen
200g (7oz) soft red fruit, cleaned and frozen (reserve some for garnish)
200g (7oz) ripe mango flesh, diced and frozen
soya milk
10ml (2 tbs) sugar-free cherry jam
10ml (2 tbs) arrowroot
1/2 pint water

Method
Heat jam and water. Make a smooth paste with the arrowroot and add to
the jam mixture. Simmer until thickened. Allow to cool before spooning
into sundae glasses. Place half the frozen bananas in a food processor
with the soft fruit, soya milk and blend. Return to freezer and blend
remaining bananas and mango. Spoon alternate layers of yellow and
pink ice cream into the sundae glasses on top of the sauce. Decorate
with toasted flaked almonds and some of the soft fruit. Serves 6.

CHOCOLATE CAKE
Ingredients
14oz (400g) dark chocolate
10oz (300g) unsalted butter
2 tbs cognac (or liqueur of your choice)
7 eggs

1 orange, lemon or lime
4 teaspoons strong coffee
1/4 cup of flour

Method
Mix the chocolate, broken into pieces, half a cup of coffee and liqueur
and melt in the top of a double boiler. Add the zest of your chosen fruit
once it has cooled. Gradually add the flour into the beaten eggs and
carefully combine the two liquids. Pour into a non-stick tin or one lined
with buttered greaseproof paper and bake in a fairly hot oven for
approximately 35-40 minutes. Serve with low-cal custard, yoghurt or a
fresh fruit puree.

FRESH ORANGE CAKE
(This is also one you will either have to wait for or allow yourself only
the teeniest morsel!)
Ingredients
200g (7oz) self-raising flour
pinch salt
100g (4oz) butter
200g (7oz) caster sugar
finely grated rind 1 orange
juice 1 orange
2 large eggs
1-2 tbs milk to mix
1 orange garnish

Method
Cream the butter. Add half the sugar and grated orange rind and beat
until soft and light. Sift the flour and salt and set aside. Lightly beat
the eggs and mix in a little at a time. Using a metal spoon, fold in the
remaining flour and a little milk to make a soft, dropping consistency.
Spoon the mixture into a greased 8" cake tine and bake in the centre of
a moderate oven for 30 minutes until risen and lightly brown. Put
strained orange juice into a pan with the sugar and heat until dissolved.
Prick the hot cake all over with a skewer and spoon the orange syrup

over the entire surface. Leave until cold. Dredge with icing sugar or cover with whipping cream and decorate with fresh orange sections for dessert. Calories? Don't ask! Serves 8-10.

ALSO AVAILABLE ON AUDIO TAPE

Paul McKenna's
STOP SMOKING FOR GOOD
This audio tape has been developed using the very latest
and most powerful hypnotic techniques to stop you smoking forever. Hypnosis is now statistically the most effective
way to give up smoking, and through this tape Paul
McKenna helps you stop smoking the easy way, leaving
you healthier, calmer and happier. The trance section of this
tape can be listened to whenever you want a boost of will
power and will effectively retrain your unconscious mind
permanently so that you too can STOP SMOKING FOR
GOOD.

Paul McKenna's
ELIMINATE STRESS
This tape combines powerful hypnotic suggestions with the
very latest techniques of personal enhancement. Using this
tape will instil a feeling of calm when dealing with even the
most hectic of schedules. ELIMINATE STRESS will transform your life into one of peace and inner strength. The
hypnotic trance section installs into your unconscious all
the resources needed to deal with a busy lifestyle. Use
ELIMINATE STRESS the natural way to a calmer, more
efficient life.

Each tape is only £9.99 (plus £1 p&p) and available from
Paul McKenna, PO Box 4RS, London W1A 4RS.

ALSO AVAILABLE ON AUDIO TAPE

Paul McKenna's
SLEEP LIKE A LOG

If insomnia is your problem use this tape and change your life. SLEEP LIKE A LOG contains the most effective techniques of hypnotherapy to give you nights of deep, refreshing sleep. The powerful hypnotic section will automatically install suggestions that will work when you need them most, ensuring a good night's sleep all night, every night.

Paul McKenna's
SUPREME SELF-CONFIDENCE

This powerful audio tape will automatically improve your self-image, making you feel more assertive and resourceful in even the most difficult situation. The hypnotic section retrains your unconscious mind, giving you a feeling of self-confidence and inner certainty you didn't know was possible. Using SUPREME SELF-CONFIDENCE regularly will change your life by teaching you how to be confident and self-assured the easy way.

Each tape is only £9.99 (plus £1 p&p) and available from Paul McKenna, PO Box 4RS, London W1A 4RS.